Klaus Oberbeil

10 Years Younger in 30 Days

Klaus Oberbeil Publishing, Inc.

All rights reserved. No part of this book may be reproduced or transmitted in any form or by any means, electronic or mechanical, including photocopying, recording, or by any information storage and retrieval system, without written permission from the publisher.

The suggestions contained in this book are not intended to replace the services of trained health professionals. All matters regarding your health require medical supervision. Recommendations presented in this book are intended for education only and not to be considered as a substitute for consultation with a duly licensed health professional. Any applications of the treatments set forth in this book are at the reader's discretion.

10 YEARS YOUNGER IN 30 DAYS

Copyright © 2005, 1999 by Klaus Oberbeil Publishing, Inc.

ISBN 0-9770905-0-7

Library of Congress Control Number: 2005931288

Cover design: Compositions/Bookmasters, Inc.
Cover photo: Banana Stock

Printed in the United States of America

Published by Klaus Oberbeil Publishing, Inc., Dover, Delaware 19901

TABLE OF CONTENTS

It's So Easy to Be Young and Beautiful 9

10 Secrets for Youthful Connective Tissue 11
  1. It's Not Always a Skin Problem 12
  2. What You Should Do When Your Connective Tissues Urgently Need Help 13
  3. There Is a Secret Life Within Our Connective Tissue That Helps Us Become, and Stay, Young 15
  4. The Cellulite Problem 18
  5. The Smoker's Dilemma 20
  6. The Beauty Inside You 22
  7. The Enemies of Your Connective Tissues 24
  8. Your Collagen Needs Rest and Sleep 26
  9. Your Connective Tissue Wants to Be Stressed and Exercised 27
  10. Your Collagen Likes It Both Ways—Warm and Cold 29

10 Secrets for Beautiful Skin 31
  11. Your Skin Is Unlike Any of Your Other Organs 32
  12. Your Skin Produces Its Own Moisture Cream 33
  13. We Would Dry Out in Less Than an Hour Without the Epidermis 35
  14. Your Skin Craves Sulfur 37
  15. Biotin Is Another Valuable Aid in Developing a Lovely Complexion 39
  16. There Is a Great Love Affair Between Your Skin and the Sun 41
  17. Secrets of a Beautiful Suntan 43
  18. Healthy Blood Circulation Makes Your Skin Look Young 45
  19. Information Regarding Psoriasis 47
  20. Create Fantastic Natural Skin Cosmetics 49

10 Secrets for Perfect Hair and Nails 53
  21. The Miracle of Your Hair 54
  22. Important Secrets Concerning Your Hair 56
  23. Your Hair Does Not Want You to Protect It—It Wants to Protect You 58
  24. The Nutrients Your Hair Needs 61
  25. Chase Off Free Radicals from Your Hair Cells 63
  26. Retain, or Even Restore, Your Natural Hair Color 65
  27. Silky, Smooth, Fuller Hair—and No Dandruff: How to Wash Your Hair .. 67
  28. Your Hair Wants to Be Prehistoric—It Does Not Want to Be Pampered .. 69
  29. Brittle Nails—Why? 71
  30. What Your Nails Need 73

The Perfect 30-Day Program for Strong Bones and Teeth 77
31. Bones Often Complain—and We Don't Listen to Them 78
32. Swallowing Calcium Tablets Is the Worst Thing You Can Do 80
33. The Nutrients Your Skeleton Needs 82
34. How the Sun Can Determine the Strength of Your Bones 84
35. Osteoporosis Is a Bone Problem Afflicting Mostly Women 86
36. Put Stress on Your Bones—They'll Like It. 88
37. Strengthen Your Skeleton with Weights 90
38. How to Rejuvenate Your Joints 92
39. Teeth: Gain Admiration and Influence People with Those Pearly Whites . . 94
40. Strong Gums for Health and Beauty 99

Lose Weight the Natural Way in One Month 101
41. Forget About All the Diet Quackery and Empty Promises 102
42. How Do People Get Fat? 104
43. The Worst Thing You Can Do Is to Eat Fat,
    Sugar-laden Foodstuffs, and White Flour Products Together 106
44. Growth Hormone Has Been Nature's Most Important Fat-Burner
    for Hundreds of Millions of Years 108
45. Other Perfect Fat-Burners: Sun, Iodine, and Fruit 112
46. Calorie-Reduced Diets Tend to Make One Fatter, Not Slimmer 114
47. A One-Way Street Named Fat 116
48. Insulin: The Fat Tyrant 118
49. How Does Physical Activity Help in the Removal of Fat Cells? 120
50. What to Eat, What to Avoid 122

Psyche and Nerves: How to Become a Happier Person in One Month . . . 125
51. Your Genetic Happiness Code 126
52. What Makes People Uneasy, Fearful, and Even Desperate 128
53. Feed Your Brain and Make Your Nerves Happy 130
54. Step Number Two: Relax Your Nerve Cells 133
55. Happiness Rises Out of Tiny Nerve-cell Vesicles 136
56. Meditating Like the Animals 140
57. In the Paradise of Sleep 142
58. How to Become a Winner 144
59. How About Emulating Einstein? 146
60. Bright Light and the Copper Enemy in Your Brain 148

Make Life More Attractive with Exercise and Physical Fitness 151
61. The Fabulous Muscles You Possess 152
62. Tell Me More About My Muscles 154
63. More Oxygen Makes You Feel More Adventuresome. 157
64. Iron Is Crucial for Your Personal Fitness 159
65. Use Your Little Stringent Factors for Better Shape 161
66. How to Build up Muscle Mass 163
67. Water—A Nutrient for Better Fitness 166
68. Learn to Walk Properly 168
69. Running Is an Excellent Exercise for All the Muscles in Your Body 170
70. Swimming Is the Second Best Exercise 172

The Exciting Experience of Regaining Youth: a 30-Day Program 175
71. Becoming Older Has Nothing to Do with Your Wall Calendar 176
72. Homocysteine Can Make You Older Than You Are 178
73. Why the "Good" Methionine Is of Such Enormous Importance
    for Your Youthful Complexion 180
74. How to Crank Up Your Methionine Score 182
75. Beware of Free Radicals 185
76. How to Protect Yourself Against Free Radicals 188
77. Nucleotides—The Building Blocks of Youth 191
78. Aging of the Brain 193
79. The Sun Is a Potent Youth Maker 196
80. Set Up New Goals 198

Your Heart and Your Circulation: Make Them More Powerful 201
81. What You Should Know About Your Heart 202
82. Your Fascinating Circulation 204
83. Another Miracle: The Blood Flowing Through Your Body 206
84. Something New About Cholesterol 208
85. Hypertension and Atherosclerosis 211
86. Hypotension: When Blood Pressure Is too Low 213
87. Why Do So Many People Neglect Their Veins? 215
88. No One Must Have Varicose Veins 217
89. Activate Your Blood Flow 219
90. Additional Ways to Help Your Circulation 221

The Wonderland of Our Organs and Our Digestion 223
91. Health and Your Intestines 224
92. Your Stomach Is a Heavy Worker 226
93. Your Intestine Is a Lush Amazon Jungle 228
94. When Cells Are Hungry 231
95. Your Liver: The Fabulous Factory Within You 233
96. Something New About Your Kidneys 235
97. Your Poor Pancreas 237
98. Make a Fortress Out of Your Immune System 239
99. Instinct: What We Can Learn from Animals and Plants 242

The Great and Novel Nutrition Plan for the New Millenium 245

Hands Off These 30 "Bad Boys" 246

Help Yourself with These Good 30 247

10 Recommended Breakfasts 248

Recommended Lunch Ingredients 249

10 Recommended Dinners 250

The Healthiest Snacks 251

Index 252

*For Monika, my beloved companion,
who made everything perfect as I wrote this book*

It's So Easy to Be Young and Beautiful

All plants and free-living animals remain young and beautiful almost to the end of their lives. All birds, fish, and deer keep their beautiful feathers, fur, or scales until just a few days, or even hours, before they die. Under a microscope the cells of a very old deer appear to be as healthy and uninjured as the body cells of a fawn.

But what a difference in the appearance of human cells! The body cells of an 18-year-old girl appear lush and gorgeous under the merciless eye of a modern, high-tech microscope. Conversely, the cells of a 45-year-old woman appear pathetically flabby and shriveled. How can youthfulness and beauty emerge out of such hopelessly faded building blocks of life?

Mother Nature wants every man, woman, and child to be as vibrantly healthy as plants and animals. Why? Because Mother Nature knows that only strong and healthy creatures reproduce strong and healthy genes and chromosomes into hundreds and thousands of future generations. This is the way all forms of life remain forever lush and beautiful, exciting and grandiose.

Nature imprinted a genetic slim-and-youth program into every one of us to guarantee this delightful evolution. Half of the roughly 80,000 active genes in the nuclei of our seventy trillion cells work day and night on the repair, maintenance, and rejuvenation of our cells. Only healthy cells promise beautiful teeth, eyes, complexion, happiness, vitality, and youthfulness.

Plants and animals almost always use up to one hundred percent of their genetic potential. They nourish themselves properly and live accordingly to the genetic rules established in their cell nucleus. A nettle plant or an ant nourishes itself and develops like its ancestors hundreds of thousands of years ago.

It is exactly this fascinating promise of Mother Nature that can be realized by everyone. *There is a younger, slimmer, more dynamic, and happier being within every man, woman, and child. All you have to do is unlock the secrets of Mother Nature's plan for beauty and youth.*

It is so incredibly easy! Genetic biologists and cell researchers have discovered a simple, but effective, program. A cell metabolism that merely operates at 50, 60, or 80 percent can never make a person vital and optimistic. So why not increase your cell metabolism to 100 percent, like animals and plants?

Follow the ninety-nine secrets for perfect beauty found within this book. You can start an entirely new life within thirty days. Seventy trillion well-nourished, happy, and eager cells will then be ready to create the new you!

10 SECRETS FOR YOUTHFUL CONNECTIVE TISSUE

1 It's Not Always a Skin Problem

People very often think that their skin is aging when wrinkles and crow's feet develop, when the tissues of the neck, breasts, belly, buttocks, or thighs become shriveled and unsightly, or when ugly cellulite turns the mirror into their personal enemy.

However, it is not primarily the skin that is weakened. It is merely that the skin lacks padding and upholstering connective tissue, or collagen. The skin regains its natural beauty when connective tissue is restored. This may happen in just a few weeks, or within a few days. Everyone knows that he or she appears, often inexplicably, younger or older on some days, or times of the day, than at others.

Why does our complexion seem to change so often? Sometimes, it changes even from one hour to the other. Why is it we go to bed with unsightly wrinkles on our cheeks and under the eyes and wake up in the morning with a smooth, more attractive complexion?

It is because our connective tissue is repaired and rejuvenated while we sleep. The condition of the skin remains the same, but not more than half a millimeter beneath the epidermis (the protecting upper skin layer), the collagen, and elastin fibers of the connective tissue have been rebuilt by trillions and trillions of microscopic enzymes.

Secret No. 1

It is very often weak connective tissue that makes us appear older than we would like.

2 What You Should Do When Your Connective Tissues Urgently Need Help

There are eight different kinds of collagen in our body for bones, organs, skin, and blood vessels, but they are all rejuvenated and exhausted in the same manner. It is important to remember that during the day, while we are working, sitting, standing, and walking, the connective tissue becomes stressed and the unbreakable netting of long protein molecules and elastic fibers often becomes very weak.

Always keep in mind that 100,000 years ago, our ancestors never worked more than about three hours a day. The rest of the day was spent just hanging around, joking, or playing with the kids—and not one of our 80,000 active genes (the managers of our entire cell metabolism) has since changed. That means that our connective tissue is as stressed as a forty year old Studebaker at full throttle going thousands of miles from Chicago to Padres Obispo, Mexico, without taking a break.

Just in time for the beginning of the new millennium, scientists discovered something amazing and extremely helpful for everyone who wants to turn back his individual biological clock—six months, two years, five years, or even more. Our connective tissue not only gives our body strength and resilience, but also provides 25 percent of our organism's protein reserve. That means that whenever our body lacks amino acids (the tiny protein building blocks), it ravenously devours them out of its own collagen, from the tip of the nose all the way down to the big toe.

That is the reason why so many people are so concerned about what they perceive to be a skin condition. In fact, it is their poor, abused collagen that is being repeatedly consumed again and again, twenty four hours a day—every hour, minute, and even second—just because seventy trillion cells are not being sufficiently nourished with essential amino acids.

Our collagen starts taking a vacation as soon as we fall asleep. What a pleasant and relaxing environment—it is so rejuvenating! There's nobody bothering us and, most importantly, nobody stealing urgently needed amino acids from you. It is during this time of the day that the amino acids work hard to make you more attractive, giving you a beautiful, healthy, and vibrant complexion.

Tiny enzymes busily knot large protein molecules together, weaving and welding them together with strong elastin fibers in collagen tissues. All this is done as you are getting your beauty sleep.

What a fulfilling life it is for a collagen enzyme to work on such an important assignment! Oh, we are all so happy helping this human become younger and much more attractive!

Secret No. 2

Skin becomes old and collagen loses vitality when our organism lacks all the amino acids needed in order to keep vital and essential organs functioning. These organs include the heart, liver, brain, and kidneys.

3 There Is a Secret Life Within Our Connective Tissue That Helps Us Become, and Stay, Young

Our stomach is flatter and stronger when we get out of bed in the morning than in the late evening, when for the last time of the day, we expose it to the bathroom mirror. The same thing happens to our face, to the skin of the neck and breast, to our buttocks and thighs, and even to our upper arms. The more we support this nightly process of rejuvenation, the more enthusiastically we can confront the mirror in the morning.

Of the twenty different amino acids in our daily nutrition, two specific ones are needed for the construction of new and young connective tissue: proline and glycine. Quadrillions of these protein building blocks flow out of the nutrition mush in the intestines through mucous membranes into the blood, and are then carried to wherever collagen is in the body.

Billions of fibroblasts (collagen-synthesizing cells) crave them. Proline and glycine are their favorite dishes, like a superb Italian tiramisu or a delicious prime rib steak would be for most of us. The very skillful fibroblasts collect these amino acids out of the supplying blood and nestle together around one thousand of them, forming one protein molecule. These molecules are tied into long fibers and then are netted. The fibers are welded together with extremely sturdy and robust elastin fibers of pure protein to make the tissue even more resilient. That way healthy collagen builds up at night and supplies our excellent fibroblasts with all the necessary raw material they need.

Amino acids are high on the list of raw materials lacking in many people who consider themselves to be aging too quickly. There is a big difference between protein in our nutrition and its smallest building blocks, the amino acids. In other words, it is difficult for our stomach and our intestines to disassemble nutrition protein—for instance out of a good bite of Thanksgiving turkey—so completely that nothing will be left other than these microscopic amino acids.

Reducing Proteins Down to Amino Acids

❉ *Most people after the age of thirty-five do not produce enough stomach acid essential to dissolve the stringy protein in their diet. That is why Mother Nature made the stomach acid of a healthy human being so acidic that it could easily burn a big hole into a valuable Persian rug in his or her living room.*

❉ *All the nutrition protein not dissolved will rot and putrefy in your lower intestines, causing indigestion symptoms such as diarrhea, flatulence, and constipation if you lack sufficient stomach acid. What is even worse is that your seventy trillion body cells are insufficiently supplied with amino acids—and will rid these essential building blocks out of your wonderful connective tissue.*

❉ *Above all, this means that you should increase the amount of stomach acid. You can do this very easily by drinking a little lemon juice or apple vinegar dissolved in water right before you start to eat your main meal. Cells in your stomach mucosa will then produce plenty of hydrochloric acid and be mixed with your gastric juices to create gastric acid.*

❉ *There will be an enormous influx of amino acids into your body metabolism—and especially into the craving fibroblasts of your connective tissues within just thirty or forty minutes after the meal. Check it out yourself: Your face may appear a lot healthier and younger within twenty-four hours.*

Supplying your collagen with the amino acids proline and glycine is not all that is needed to create new connective tissues. Netting unbreakable collagen together is not an easy job for your fibroblasts while you are sleeping. In addition, they need the trace element zinc and plenty of vitamin C. Both are essential as enzyme donors, the tiny "elves" which do all the real work at night.

Take diluted lemon juice or apple vinegar one or two minutes before you start eating your main meals in order to develop more of these amino acids. Zinc is highly concentrated in oysters, liver, egg yolks, red muscle meat (steaks), lobster, and in all types of grain or cereals like wheat, rye, oat, barley, spelt, buckwheat, and millet. Want to accelerate the restoration of your collagen? Then take zinc lozenges and the white ascorbic acid powder (it is available in pharmacies, drugstores, and health shops) as daily nutrition supplements.

The more amino acids, zinc, and vitamin C you rush into your fibroblasts the more often you will hear admiring (and sometimes envious) congratulations like, "You look so young! You look ten years younger since I met you last time at Kmart. Where were you on vacation?"

Secret No. 3

Help your fibroblasts restore youthful collagen overnight. All they need are more amino acids, zinc, and vitamin C.

4 The Cellulite Problem

Cellulite is not at all a skin problem—it is a connective tissue problem.

You may massage, knead, and rub creams into the skin of your thighs, follow all the good (or not-so-good) advice of mail-order frauds, and it all will not help. Why don't animals suffer from cellulite? Because they properly live and nourish themselves correctly.

So, why not learn from them? Nothing is easier than that.

Cellulite is a problem for women. Women genetically accumulate fat more easily than men. Women need and deposit more fat than men for the protection and nutrient support of their growing babies.

The epidermis (the upper skin layer) of women is in most cases thinner than the one found in men. Their fat cells in the dermis (which is beneath the epidermis) are—unlike men—separated by very weak walls. Their partition walls are thin and vulnerable. The fat cells of women, particularly within the skin of their thighs or buttocks, are bigger. What makes it worse is that they stand upright and develop like bolts. The more fat that women collect within in the adipocytes (fat cells) and fat tissues of their thighs and buttocks, the more these overdeveloped fat-bolts push against the thin upper epidermis, causing it to elevate. The symptoms of the so-called orange skin appear as the number of these protrusions increase.

Do Not Ever Attempt to Use Slimming "Cures" for Cellulite

❋ *Slimming cures only cause the thin connective tissue to become even weaker. The bolt-like pressure of the hard fat cells against the epidermis builds up, and the cellulite condition becomes worse.*

❋ *The first step in reducing or eliminating cellulite is to fortify and strengthen the connective tissue.*

❋ *The second step is to reduce body fat. How that efficiently works (thanks to the twenty-first century research of cell researchers and molecular biologists) will be presented later in this book.*

Secret No. 4

You can eliminate your cellulite problem by strengthening your connective tissue.

5 The Smoker's Dilemma

Granted, it is difficult for some people to stop smoking. It is difficult just to cut down from twenty to ten and from ten to just four or five a day. Some people are stressed from early morning to late at night—taking care of the kids and the husband or wife, hustling to work, doing the housework, and dealing with daily problems. So why not a couple of cigarettes a day?

It is not healthy at all, physicians say. They are, of course, right. Smoking is not only a physical addiction, but also a psychological addiction. Many attempt to relieve their stress levels by lighting up. This satisfies the individual for only a short period of time because his or her body craves nicotine.

Cigarettes are not healthy, whether it is in the form of a physical or psychological addiction. They are nutrient robbers. Every cigarette robs the body of twenty-five milligrams of important vitamin C because all the poisonous tar and nicotine in a cigarette has to be unconditionally neutralized by the immune system. It is poison, pure poison. Mother Nature would have grown cigarettes in woods and fields if cigarettes were healthy. Foxes, deer, eagles, and buffaloes would be walking a mile for a Camel and lighting up after creating an offspring if cigarettes were healthy.

I am sorry to rain on your parade by pointing out that cigarettes extensively damage your health. However, in spite of the indisputable facts that cigarettes cause serious health problems there are millions of smokers, even heavy smokers.

We have read that vitamin C is vital for the creation of youthful connective tissue. It is no wonder that some smokers develop plenty of tiny wrinkles above their upper lip and under their eyes. The reason is because the immune system needs all the vitamin C contained in the daily nutritional intake to immunologically rid itself of the tar and nicotine poison. The connective tissue is insufficiently supplied with the important enzyme donor for the maintenance of collagen.

Therefore, it should be clear that smokers require increased quantities of vitamin C.

Smokers should start the day with a fruit breakfast. One banana, a kiwi, and half an apple cut into pieces, with cream and a tablespoon of sunflower kernels and perhaps a glass of fresh-pressed orange juice can ward off much of the harmful effects of a couple of cigarettes a day.

If your connective tissues could talk, they would thank you because they really need that vitamin C—to make you look youthful and beautiful.

Secret No. 5

Smokers should consume more vitamin C—that means plenty of fresh fruit and vitamin C tablets as supplements.

6 The Beauty Inside You

Common knowledge has it that if you are beautiful outside, you are also beautiful inside and vice versa. If you suffer from bleeding gums, you also bleed inside because your vessels are weak. More precisely, that means the walls of your veins and arteries are undernourished.

If your internal body lacks amino acids, your face, your cheeks, your breasts, your neck, and elsewhere will lack protein in the form of amino acids as well.

Here is one example: glycosaminoglycans—a complicated word, which only scientists are able to create. These molecules are beauty molecules. The more you collect these beauty molecules the younger you are. Glycosaminoglycans hold all the necessary water within your collagen. Your collagen will shrink if it lacks water. Amino acids such as proline and glycine, trace elements such as zinc, and a thousand vitamin C-rich apples will not help.

If you are well nourished, the connective tissue within you will always be ecstatic: "We are so happy, so unbelievably happy!" Your connective tissue also recognizes that it requires water.

Try it out yourself right this minute: press your finger against your cheek. If your tissue snaps back like rubber, your collagen is in fine condition. This demonstrates that connective tissues need water for that particular purpose.

Glycosaminoglycans retain that important water. All the collagen fibers are embedded in these important molecules. There are several types of basic substances for all of your youthful connective tissues. Please read more about them in the following chapters about beautiful skin.

You know that the tank of your car is useless without gas. The same thing is true with all the marvelous glycosaminoglycans in your connective tissue. Water is what they need and what they urgently request. Many people complain of shriveled skin—and do not know that all the connective tissue in their body is flabby as well. The simple reason is that they do not drink enough. The older you become, the more fluid your body, particularly your collagen, needs. Get used to drinking more, much more, fluids in the form of fruit and vegetable juice (self-pressed juices are the best), water, mineral water, and black or green tea.

Your visible connective tissue will express its appreciation by releasing the secret beauty within you. You will never again recognize your collagen.

Secret No. 6

Drink more fluids. Not only will your connective tissues thank you, but your internal organs as well.

7 The Enemies of Your Connective Tissues

Free radicals are enemies of unhealthy connective tissues.

Many people think free radicals are nothing but unwelcome news because of what they have read in newspapers and magazines.

Free radicals are not entirely bad, though they are inexorable enemies of our connective tissue and of our entire organism as well.

Roughly 500 million years ago, Mother Nature said, "All I want on earth are healthy, vibrant plants and creatures. Only they can guarantee the continuation and development of healthy races and families of all my beautiful plants and beings."

Therefore, Mother Nature invented the free radicals. She told them, "The only job you have on earth is killing everything that is sick or apparently unable to live well." When autumn comes we see a leaf circling down from a tree, one half faded and withered, and the other half still young and green. If we were to return to that leaf, sometime later, we would see that the entire leaf would be brown and dead. The free radicals have killed the surviving green plant cells. Mother Nature says, "Good work, guys. You've done your job well."

Free radicals are very aggressive molecules, destroying every plant, animal, or human cell that is weak and vulnerable. However, they are not at all bad. They are not offended or annoyed at all whenever they are confronted with a healthy and protected human cell. They just back off and seek other victims.

So, as long as we keep our connective tissue immune protected, free radicals would rather be our friends and not do our collagen any harm.

There are four protecting substances our collagen needs to stay young and healthy. They are the vitamins A, C, and E and the trace element selenium. Vitamin A, or its precursors, the carotenes, are highly concentrated in all green, yellow, and red fruits and vegetables such as apricots, peaches, pumpkin, melons, red or dark berries, paprika, tomatoes, spinach, carrots, cabbage, broccoli, leek, chard, salad greens, green peas, green beans, avocados, and in liver. Fresh fruits contain plenty of vitamin C, especially acidic fruits like kiwi, grapefruit, lemons, and sour apples. All plant oils are rich in vitamin E. Selenium is highly concentrated in all grains or cereals, as well as natural rice, mushrooms, asparagus, garlic, cheese, eggs, and liver.

These four antioxidants are also available in pharmacies, drugstores, and health-stores.

Secret No. 7

Protect your vulnerable connective tissue with the wonderful helpers: A, C, E, and selenium.

8 Your Collagen Needs Rest and Sleep

Why do we recover during sleep? Our bodies are invigorated after sleeping because circulation, heartbeat, and brain waves slow down, while the intestines increase their activities. They deliver substantial amounts of nutrients through their mucosa into the blood for further transport to the cells. The delivered nutrients include vitamins, minerals, trace elements, fatty acids, glucose, amino acids, and nucleic acids. The cells—and particularly those of the connective tissue—receive replacements for what they gave away during the day. This means that rest and sleep are important factors for recovering and rejuvenating your collagen. While you are still up in the evening or even at night, your seventy trillion body cells claim all the nutrients transported in your blood—and that makes your collagen run down.

In addition, there is another reason why sleep is so important for your beauty and complexion. Your immune system and your collagen are, in a way, twins. They both lose substance during the day and can only regain it and recover during rest or sleep.

Read more about your restoring immune system and rejuvenating sleep in following chapters.

Secret No. 8

Every minute of rest or sleep is invaluable help for the restoration of your connective tissue.

9 Your Connective Tissue Wants to Be Stressed and Exercised

Sitting in your fine high-backed easy chair, doing nothing, will not do your collagen any good. Mother Nature would have all her wonderful animals just sit around out there in the woods and the fields if it were so. Collagen wants to work, it wants to demonstrate how unbreakable and sturdy and attractive it is.

Scientists have compared connective tissue cells of zoo animals with those of free-living birds and monkeys. What a difference! The collagen of even young caged birds and zoo monkeys was poor, flabby, and faded when compared to that of the free-living birds and animals. It's no wonder that such a condition exists when a sad parrot has nothing to do except to perch on his swing all day. So, his collagen cells keep saying, "Why should we make an effort in being strong and attractive? Our master, the parrot, is happy and satisfied on that ridiculous swing all day."

Any kind of physical exercise supplies each of your connective tissue cells with power, vitality, and energy. Exercise, even for just a few minutes, throttles up the cell metabolism to 100 percent. The best thing to do is drink the juice of one grapefruit and immediately after take a five minute walk or jog in fresh air. You can also practice your indoor sports. Open the window and jump trampoline, do situps, stretching exercises, aerobics, or whatever you would like. Your collagen cells will say, "Thank you, thank you very much!" A little exercise is they want and need.

Secret No. 9

From now on, ride the elevators and escalators only when going downstairs— never upstairs.

10 Your Collagen Likes it Both Ways—Warm and Cold

We can learn so much from free-living plants and animals, even from the most seemingly insignificant weed beside the road. Animals and plants use temperature changes for genetic vitality impulses and so can we.

We can only roughly estimate the temperature by saying that it is 62 or 64 degrees. Our skin knows better. It is an extremely sensitive antenna. It reacts on temperature changes within a hundredth of a degree. It reports the slightest changes to the nerves and the brain, which in turn stimulate cells and tissue, especially our collagen.

Our connective tissue has not changed for 100,000 or 200,000 years. It has evolved after being exposed to the sun and the storm, the snow and the heat, the rain and the frost, and the fog and the warmth. It has been trained by temperature changes—and it likes it that way.

Our grandma lectured us, "When we were young, the kitchen was marvelously warm and cozy. The hall and even the living room were chilly, and not very inviting. In addition, the toilets were so terribly icy cold. We would try to stay in the kitchen as long as possible."

In addition, these temperature changes are exactly what our connective tissues—and our skin—like the most. Establish "climate zones" in your home. When you go for a walk, do not dress too warmly. Let the skin and the connective tissues of your face learn to love the cold. Never heat up your bedroom like a factory stove.

Secret No. 10

Take one or two cold/hot showers a day. Your connective tissue will love it.

You Can Have Young and Strong Connective Tissue Within 30 Days

- *Supply your collagen with many more amino acids by drinking lemon juice or apple vinegar before the main meals.*

- *Eat plenty of vitamin C-rich fresh fruit.*
  Take zinc lozenges for 30 days.

- *Avoid junk food; eat more legumes and vegetables.*

- *Cut down on smoking.*

- *Drink more—your connective tissue needs fluid.*

- *Take antioxidant drugs for 30 days.*

- *Rest or sleep one more hour than you are used to doing.*

- *Exercise daily—and if it is just for five minutes, twice a day.*

- *Expose your skin to cold or chill at least once a day.*

- *Change the temperature from hot to cold several times while you are under the shower.*

10 SECRETS FOR BEAUTIFUL SKIN

11 Your Skin Is Unlike Any of Your Other Organs

Yes, the skin is an organ, too, and built up in three layers: 1) the epidermis which does not contain blood vessels is 0.1 millimeter thick, 2) the dermis beneath which is rich in connective tissue, and 3) the inner layer which mainly consists of connective tissue and fat is up to 25 millimeters thick. The skin is our largest and heaviest organ. It makes up 15 percent of our body weight.

A little spot on the skin of your face, not bigger than the nail of your thumb, contains 1 yard of blood vessels, 120 sweat glands, about 20 oil and 50 follicle glands, 5 yards of nerve fibers, thousands of pigment cells (which are important for an attractive suntan; read about that later), 2 yards of lymph vessels, and about 30 nerve endings for your sense of touch and your sense of pain. Every day your skin sweats out up to 2 liters of fluid, or even more when it is extremely hot.

Your skin has to manage an extraordinarily complex and difficult job because it is the border and the connection to the outer world. The skin protects us against heat, cold, sunbeams, bacteria, and other pathogenic microorganisms. Moreover, the skin manages the contact to our environment—even if such contact means painful cuffs, pokes, or scratches.

Secret No. 11

Your skin lives permanently on the frontier. It protects you. Give it some protection, too.

12 Your Skin Produces Its Own Moisture Cream

Your skin creates the best moisture creams available—better than anything you can buy in a beauty shop or drugstore.

An unconditional battle is raging wherever you look. Battles like that are also being carried out on your skin. Millions and millions of bacteria, fungi, viruses, parasites, and other microbes are struggling to somehow enter your body.

In order to ward them off, our skin produces a very fine protecting film which is so acidic that it kills hostile microorganisms or at least frightens them off. That, incidentally, is the reason why our skin tastes a little bit acidic.

The skin fills this film with its own troops in order to build up an even stronger bastion. It does so by infusing its own "good" bacteria and fungi. These are very well armed and trained to kill the invading enemies who do not have good intentions in our body. By being so well protected, our skin is virtually immune against pathogenic microbes and we will not very easily contract skin diseases.

These are reasons enough not to destroy your own protecting skin film with the wrong soaps, cleansers, creams, ointments, liniments, and tinctures. Your skin will never accept these. The wrong cleansing cream may demonstrate its supposed cleansing "quality" when your cotton swab appears soiled. Actually, most of this "dirt" is your wonderful protection film: old sweat deposits, rancid sebum, dead protein garbage and dead skin scales—altogether a perfectly organized environment for your own "good" bacteria and parasites in which to live.

Be sure your next cleanser or soap is skin friendly. You should ask your pharmacist or the sales staff in a reputable beauty shop.

Secret No. 12

Your skin produces its own superior moisture and protection film. Never wash it off with an inferior cleanser.

13 We Would Dry Out in Less Than an Hour Without the Epidermis

This outer scaly layer is impenetrable for most pathogenic substances. It is like a concrete wall and is, at the same time, soil for an extremely rich microflora of "good" viruses, bacteria, yeast, and mites. A scientist once determined that there are more than 700,000 of these protecting microbes in just one square centimeter. That is unbelievable!

The scale-building cells, keratinocytes, are rather intelligent. They recognize hostile microorganisms and respond with the production of certain immune substances such as interleukin. The keratinocytes activate lymphocytes that may give rise to inflammations. That, for example, may happen after a gnat bite. The inflammation then struggles against the intruding poison. That is one good reason why you should take care of your epidermis.

Though your epidermis does not contain blood vessels, it is highly dependent on healthy nutrition. Otherwise, this skin layer will no longer be able to absorb water. A healthy and well-nourished epidermis can absorb three times its body weight in water.

Your epidermis will be undernourished if you eliminate fruit, vegetables, grain, and other healthy food from your diet. It also loses the fantastic ability of absorbing much water and the ability to produce its own moisturizing cream.

Even worse is the fact that the epidermis also loses the ability to retain body water and its contribution to the body's water regulation and maintenance. You start sweating too much—and your body loses water. That weakens your connective tissue, your muscles, and your glands, making you appear older than you are.

Your epidermis develops its resiliency from its metabolism, never externally. It does so although it consists almost entirely of dead-scale cells called keratin. It is highly dependent on healthy food—more than you would ever think.

Secret No. 13

Your intestines will allow you to develop a youthful outer skin layer, but only if you eat right.

14 Your Skin Craves Sulfur

There are twenty amino acids within the epithel of the epidermis other than your connective tissue that consists mainly of just two amino acids: proline and glycine. One of the twenty amino acids in your outer skin layer is of special importance. It is referred to as cysteine. The protein building block transports the entire juvenile sulfur into the skin. Your skin would dry out faster than the Sahara under the blazing sun without sulfur.

Mother Nature was presented with a problem as small, and later, large animals such as dinosaurs and humans evolved. How could Mother Nature offer these creatures protection against ultraviolet light? Sulfur is one element able to do that. Sulfur contributes highly to the moisture-rich, lipid-rich outer skin barrier.

However, sulfur is also the most stubborn of all elements. Unlike almost all other elements, it never makes the slightest effort to enter body cells. Yes, sulfur is lazy, no doubt about it. In addition, it is clever. Sulfur always wants to be driven around. Moreover, it would not accept any taxi either. It only accepts luxury limousines—the amino acids methionine, taurine, and for the transport into the skin, cysteine. There is no doubt about it. Your diet must be rich in that particular protein building block. Very rich in cysteine are legumes, especially beans, soya, and tofu products; egg yolk; onions; and garlic. That is why people in sunny countries have traditionally enriched their meals with these foodstuffs for thousands and thousands of years.

Cysteine not only protects your skin from desiccation, it also makes your skin wonderfully flexible and elastic. Besides that, cysteine is part of the most effective immune molecule in your body: glutathione-peroxidase. Glutathione-peroxidase is your epidermis' stronghold against the free radicals, which are produced by the photons in the UV beams of the sun and which day by day try to harm your wonderful, youthful skin.

Do you understand now why makers of cosmetics so persistently try to push the important sulfur into your skin cells from the outside? It is not because it works, but rather it is because most people are gullible and want to believe that skin beauty must be bought off the shelves in expensive creams. These creams are ineffective and can be easily washed off in the evening.

Secret No. 14

Eat sulfur-rich food and your skin will develop a beautiful complexion.

15 Biotin Is Another Valuable Aid in Developing a Lovely Complexion

This vitamin belongs to the helpful B family and is synthesized in your intestines. You can also eat biotin-rich foods such as egg yolks; tomatoes; soya beans; natural, unprocessed rice; liver; oat flakes; carrots; and peanuts.

You can be sure of one thing when you meet a person with wonderfully silky, smooth, and beautiful skin (and hair): This person has no biotin problem. Not more than a thousandth gram, deposited in the liver, is necessary to bring the desired results. Beauty does not have to be expensive. It is easy to see that Mother Nature is still the best and least expensive beauty salon.

The same as cysteine, biotin is able to bind sulfur and carry it to the skin. It helps your skin to control the secretion of sebum, that way stopping a pathologic overproduction of the sebaceous glands. Your skin will easily become gray without biotin. It is also one of the best natural drugs against nervousness or irritability because biotin also helps establishing healthy glucose concentrations in the blood (which is a positive blood-sugar level), supporting your nerve cells with their important fuel, glucose. It is no wonder people with nervous symptoms complain about aged, gray skin.

Biotin is further proof that beauty develops from our own intestines—healthy intestines, that is. When the sensible microflora in the intestines becomes slowly destroyed by the wrong food, the bacteria in the microflora are no longer able to produce all the biotin a smooth skin needs.

In addition, biotin has powerful enemies in the wrong food including sugar, liquors, and industrially-processed grain.

The first warning symptoms of a biotin deficiency are skin scales, tiny fissures in a dry skin—an epidermis that becomes too scaly. Sooner or later skin inflammation will develop and the skin will appear withered and otherwise unhealthy.

Secret No. 15

Don't put your faith in biotin-rich cosmetics. Supply your skin with its own biotin by eating nutrient-rich food.

16 There Is a Great Love Affair Between Your Skin and the Sun

It takes a photon (part of a sunbeam) eight minutes for an adventurous 100,000 million-mile journey from the sun through cold space to your skin cells. There it immediately slips into a cholesterol-containing cell and starts working. It takes one or even two days until the tiny photon has managed to build a calciferol-molecule, precursor of life-giving vitamin D. Sunbeams are best friends whenever our skin is protected.

Now, at the beginning of the new millenium, cell researchers have discovered astonishing new facts about this hormone-like vitamin. First, it does not need any enzymes to become synthesized. Second, it is one of the very few molecules allowed to slide through the protecting membranes of all our seventy trillion cells. More than that, it also doesn't need a gate pass to enter the inner membrane around the cell nucleus right into the chromosomes and the genes, the hidden managers of our metabolism and health.

With the exception of vitamin A and thyroxine, the hormone of our thyroid gland, all other molecules are required to first approach their specific receptor at the outside of these membranes and ask "May I come in?"

Genetic researchers call vitamin D a transcription factor. It stimulates genes to release vitality impulses into every cell. That is why the sun is so essential to life, and in addition, why we feel so good when we are, or were, in the sun. Besides that, the vitamin D molecule is the instrument with which the sun still rules us, as she does with all plants and animals.

Understandably, vitamin D does the most important job within our skin cells—it keeps them busy and young. It ensures that the cell metabolism of the skin cells always reach their optimal level. Free-living animals do not have any problems with that because they always collect plenty of photons during the day.

What a difference it makes to us humans, as we are so often forced into rooms without sunlight for hours on end—sometimes the entire day. However, without these lovely tiny photons our skin cells are inactive and so very unhappy. How they yearn for just a couple of these wonderful sunbeams!

All cysteine, biotin, and any other nutrients are useless without the golden photons from the sun.

So the sun tells us, "I give them to you for free. As many as you want. Why don't you reach out and take them? Collect them and take advantage of these life-giving rays as animals and plants do."

Secret No. 16

Enjoy the sun's rays—at least once a day for 20 minutes.

17 Secrets of a Beautiful Suntan

Up to 10 percent of the cells of your skin are melanocytes. Our skin needs them in order to filter out dangerous UV beams. The more people are exposed to the sun in their original environment, the more melanocytes enriched is their skin. That is why people in Africa develop more melanocytes and have darker skin than people in the temperate climate zones.

The darker someone's skin is and the more melanocytes this skin possesses, the less he or she will suffer from sunburn. On the other hand, people with extremely light skin—such as most people with red hair—develop fewer melanocytes and are therefore especially exposed to the danger of certain UV beams. Those parts of your skin which are exposed to the sun most frequently, usually the face, neck, and hands, contain the most suntanning melanocytes. Our pituitary gland in the inner brain (the gland is not bigger than the seed of a cherry) instructs the melanocytes to synthesize their color pigment, melanin, the moment we leave the house and step into the bright sunshine.

The more intensive the sunbeams attack our skin, the more the pigment melanin is produced. The tiny melanin factories are in the lower regions of your skin. The pigment molecules slowly wander upward into the outer scaly layer of the epidermis, where they will be systematically disassembled by enzymes. That is why our marvelous vacation suntan never lasts longer than a few days. Now read what you can do for an optimal attractive suntan that lasts much longer.

In the forenoon, in the afternoon, or even in the early evening, your skin (when exposed to the sun) will develop a silky nougat or fine brown much easier than in the parching heat of noon. Why is that? Because during the afternoon hours the pituitary gland secretes less of its tanning hormone MSH (melanocyte-stimulating hormone).

MSH are tiny molecules which stimulate the synthesis of the melanin pigments.

Our skin is rather defenseless without MSH when exposed to UV beams, which are at noon up to thirty times more dangerous than in the forenoon or afternoon. In addition, what is worse is that the noon sun increases the risk of sunburn and the tan it produces will often not even last until the next morning. Overnight your skin cells will produce extreme amounts of pigment dissembling enzymes in order to get rid of this unphysiological accumulation of melanin pigments.

So in the morning, nothing will be left of that great suntan you carried around in your hotel lobby being admired by people left and right. Your skin will be scaly and insufficiently supplied with blood.

Secret No. 17

Never expose your precious skin to the sun during the noon-time, even in winter.

18 Healthy Blood Circulation Makes Your Skin Look Young

Why do our kids look so lovely when they come storming in from school or the playground? Because their skin, and particularly that of the face, is so well supplied with blood.

Some people live with a miracle. Sometimes their mirror reflects the face of an insignificant gray Cinderella; another day their face emits glowing charisma and personality you seldom see, even in the movies. Typical for those people are the ones who hang idly around on their sofa, not even reading because life is so boring. The moment the phone rings or—even better, when they are in the middle of a milling crowd of a party, with all that noise and music and talking going on—their face looks so wonderfully young. That's because there is better blood flow in their skin stimulated by hormones, neuropeptides, and neurotransmitters like ACTH, beta-endorphin, or norepinephrine.

Increased blood circulation in your face is tremendous help for anybody who wants to look more attractive. Very often, it is just a matter of improved blood flow in your face and the skin of your neck, which improves personal appearance and consequently effects personal success.

It is not only because the face looks younger; there is one more important reason. The blood system is able to bring nutrients, like vitamins, proteins, or trace elements, right into the skin of your face. In addition, these nutrients increase your skin cell metabolism and therefore create the conditions necessary to improve the skin to 100 percent metabolism in the beauty zone. It is now obvious that you should make every effort to optimize blood flow and circulation through your skin.

How do you do that? It is easier than you may think. Remember: Nature's pharmacy always works quickly, within one or two days, even within a few hours. It is not like the doctors, who tell you, "Take that pill, madam, for two or three months, and you should notice an improvement."

No, you can have a more attractive face and skin within one day if you adhere to certain rules: 1) Eat more foodstuffs containing substances that stimulate a better blood flow; and 2) Expose your skin to the interaction of hot and cold.

1) Here is what you should eat: onions, garlic, leek, paprika, peppers, fennel, radish, horseradish, celery. Drink a little apple vinegar, mixed with water, before your main meals. What you should not eat, because it makes your blood thicker are sugar, anything which is sweet (also avoid sweet drinks), white bread or grain, polished rice, fat sauces, dips, dressings, mayonnaise, or canned, instant, and microwave meals.

2) Take cold/hot showers, walk in the fresh air, and commit yourself to doing regular and vigorous exercise at least once a day. It will improve the circulation throughout your body, not just the skin of your face.

Secret No. 18

Let your face blossom again— with better circulation.

19 Information Regarding Psoriasis

About half of the patients inherit this disease from their parents. Symptoms include silver-white or white scales around slightly elevated little skin regions, mostly on the back of the hands, the knuckles, elbows, knees, and the skin of the head. Itching, burning, and inflammation are also typical symptoms. This skin problem very often breaks out from one day to the other.

The reason is that basal cells of the epidermis suddenly start dividing themselves up to 1,000 times faster than before. Scientists call that pathologic proliferation.

However, there must be also a reason for that. When we are under stress all day, badly nourished, no rest, and no sleep nor sunlight or fresh air, our immune system becomes increasingly weakened and especially the one in your skin. Because your skin cells also have to fight intruding factors like heat, cold, poisonous substances, and bacteria, they use up tremendous amounts of precious immune substances such as vitamins or certain protein molecules.

Then all of a sudden, the immune barrier of your skin breaks down—often overnight and mostly during the wet and cold winter months, when the body needs and wastes more immune substances. There is usually just one factor that causes the disease. A stressful situation such as a personal conflict, a job problem, or being the recipient of bad news can cause the outbreak of this skin disease.

Arachidonic acid, a fatty acid that is predominantly contained in meat or meat products, is a substance which promotes psoriasis. That is why heavy meat eaters more often suffer from that disease than people who favor fish or plant food. The metabolism uses arachidonic acid to synthesize leukotrienes, immune mediators, which in turn attract trillions of white immune blood cells as a seeming helpful army. Instead of doing much good, these troops finally topple the balance of your poor skin cell's immune system and that of your orderly mitosis, the cell division.

Switch from meat to fish—or better fat-containing plant food like avocado, soya, and other beans. These types of foods are synthesized into other sorts of immune mediators in your metabolism, so there is less harm and less inflammation. Your body is then supplied with omega-fatty acids, which in any case are our best friends. Therefore always try to use plant oils in your kitchen instead of any other fat.

Your skin needs UV light as well when you have psoriasis. Nucleus receptors (tiny protein molecules on the protecting membrane of the nuclei of your skin cells) catch these UV beams and use them for synthesizing a just recently discovered family of vitamin D molecules. They also block the "bad" leukotrienes, which are responsible for psoriasis.

Secret No. 19

Sun, cold-water fish, and avocadoes are powerful enemies of your psoriasis.

20 Create Fantastic Natural Skin Cosmetics

You need typical kitchen products such as mayonnaise, lemon juice, soya oil, butter, strawberries, apple vinegar, cucumbers, yogurt, egg yolk, honey, avocado, lavender, thyme, rosemary, arnica and many other herbs, sea salt, milk, self-pressed fruit juice, ginger, and vanilla, to create your own natural cosmetics.

You cannot do anything wrong by mixing up your own lotions, creams, or tinctures. The more creativity you invest, the more fun you will have. Why not supply your entire family with wonderful self-made cosmetics?

You should consider just a few things:

1) Contrary to all the cosmetics you normally buy, your natural cosmetics should be used as soon as possible, at best within a few days, or—when you keep them in your fridge—within one or two weeks. That is because nature does not preserve her products with all kinds of poisonous bacteria- and fungi-killers. Your cosmetics will become rancid or spoiled, if not used up quickly.

2) Overcome your beliefs that foodstuffs, like squashed apricots, are only to be eaten and not rubbed into one's face, or that potatoes shouldn't be put through the mixer and then put on your breasts.

3) Wash your skin thoroughly before you apply your new cosmetics. Natural substances are not as aggressive as the ones you often buy in drugstores. The pores of your skin must be clean and open to promote the absorption of all the wonderful vitamins, enzymes, or other molecules.

Secret No. 20

Let your imagination freely explore the fascinating nature's garden in order to create the finest cosmetics possible.

Make Your Skin 10 Years Younger— in Just 30 Days

- *Give your skin all the protection it needs with immune substances like vitamins A, C, and D.*

- *Never wash off the natural protection film on your skin with cheap, ineffective cleansers.*

- *Eat healthy foodstuffs. Never forget that beautiful skin originates from healthy and well-nourished intestines.*

- *Prepare meals that are rich in sulfur and biotin.*

- *Your skin loves the sun—allow it at least 20 minutes a day in bright light.*

- *Make sure that you increase circulation and blood flow in your skin.*

- *Fight psoriasis—with sunbeams, cold-water fish, and avocados.*

- *Make and use your own healthy and natural skin cosmetics.*

10 SECRETS FOR PERFECT HAIR AND NAILS

21 The Miracle of Your Hair

It is unbelievable but your hair is dead. It is made up of lifeless horn-shafts constructed of 99 percent keratin, a protein substance; some sulfur; and other ingredients such as trace elements. In spite of being dead, it can look so marvelously bustling and full of life. How is that possible?

According to the molecular structure, there is no big difference between your hair and the fur of a breathtakingly beautiful leopard or Siberian tiger. Both are merely keratin, a dead protein horn stuff.

The fact is that as long as this keratin shaft grows out of the hair follicle, it is full of lively youth, ambition, and curious about what happens outside the tight cells of that follicle. This is similar to an egg embryo, for instance of a chicken, which curiously bursts out of the shell in order to check out what life is all about.

Every single hair is a miracle—one of the most fascinating creations of Mother Nature.

A young hair shaft rises out of the skin of your head and dies. The follicle eagerly combines proteins, sulfur, and other substances together and pushes the growing hair out, day after day. The miracle is that our hair keeps its youthful beauty even from the point where it is no more than keratin. It is probably the only product of our body, which stays beautiful—dead as well as alive.

Our hair can never be beautified from outside. Sprays, conditioners, and most shampoos are ineffective. All you can do to your dead hair shafts is to cover and guard them with certain hair cosmetics that sheathe them with a fine film, protecting them from early splitting.

It is very important, if you really desire lush, silky, full, and colorful hair, to ensure that the follicles are sufficiently supplied with nutrients so they can always do their wonderful job.

Secret No. 21

The beauty of your hair starts with the follicles.

22 Important Secrets Concerning Your Hair

Healthy hair consists of between 80,000 and 120,000 strands of hair. Blonde-haired people have the most; brown-haired people have less hair, and red heads have the least.

Do not worry! Losing hair is normal. You lose approximately 100 strands of hair a day. Finding them in your comb may not be a disaster at all. The growth of our hair goes in phases. Hair keeps growing over the years and then suddenly takes a rest. No one knows why. About every seventh single hair stays in that "vacation phase." At the end of the entire period of growing and not growing, then comes the big final stop. About every hundredth of our hair is in that phase. These are the hair shafts you will find in your comb or on your shoulder.

Our hair has a life span of between one and five years. Hair shafts grow about three millimeters every ten days. The hair-producing cells of the skin of your head belong to the most active in your whole body, just exceeded in activity rates by the cells of your bones and especially the cells of the alveolar bone in the maxilla of your jaw which holds your teeth. You can read about that later as well.

Whether someone has sleek, wavy, or curly hair depends on the follicles. You cannot in any way influence that. How does the color get into your hair? Melanocytes (color-giving cells) live right in the heart of the follicles and secrete their pigments into the growing hair shaft—either black, brown, red, or blond. You cannot influence that either. Melanocytes are extremely stubborn. They act just the way they want or the way the inherited genes and chromosomes tell them.

Secret No. 22

Your hair cells are extremely productive. Supply them with all the nutrients they need and they will make you young and beautiful.

23 Your Hair Does Not Want You to Protect It—It Wants to Protect You

We visit a drugstore, supermarket, or beauty shop and we find the remedies include hair-protecting conditioners, lotions, shampoos, sprays, and strengtheners. They all promise to protect your hair.

However, our hair does not want to be protected. On the contrary, it wants to protect us—from heat or cold, fog, snow, rain, or frost. It is the same as the fur and coats of all the wonderful free-living animals. They are permanently confronted with good or bad weather, the sun, and the frost.

Each and every one of our hair follicles follows a genetic program, which has been imprinted into the chromosomes of the hair-building cells hundreds of thousand years ago, even millions of years ago, when our ancestors were chimpanzees. Our genotype, the sum of all of our genes, has since then changed just one percent. Our follicles function the same way as they did thousands of generations ago. According to our hair and their follicles, we are still apes.

That doesn't sound very encouraging, but that's the way it is. We sit in our office, in front of computers, involved with high-tech assignments, working on the most innovating challenges—and in the meantime, our hair grows exactly like the hair of apes. Can that be possible?

We should be happy and proud of that, and we should support our hair in any way we can to keep it growing like the coat of a chimpanzee. That is exactly the right way to become admired, "I wish I had that young, vibrant, luxurious hair you have. What kind of conditioner do you use?"

The year 2000 is a precursor to many exciting changes—thanks to genetic researchers, molecular biologists, neuroendocrinologists, and cell researchers. The time is in the past when pharmaceutical companies told us of chemically-synthesized drugs which were supposed to be superior to all that nature has ever given birth. The good news is that scientists are now researching the puzzles and secrets of nature. They are convinced that nature is, and remains, the best healer as well as the best pharmacist.

And what does Dr. Nature tell us? What your hair really wants you to do is to get out into the rain, without any headgear, and jog or walk for just five minutes. Return home, slightly sweating, get under the hot shower (even better would be hot/cold), rub your hair dry, and you will realize within a few minutes that it gains a strong and youthful consistency.

That is what Dr. Nature says. And how do genetic researchers explain this phenomenon? By doing this, several dozen of our 80,000 active genes, the ones which are responsible for hair growth, send stimulating impulses to the cells in the hair follicles. The cells increase their growing activities, the melanocytes secrete more color pigments into the growing hair shaft, and more smoothing sulfur will join the process.

How does all that look scientifically? The hair-growing genes transcript their code onto mRNAs—imprints of their pattern (researchers name them messenger ribonucleic acid, a terrible word). These ambitious mRNAs slip through tiny pores of the nucleus membrane into the large watery cytoplasma of the follicle cells—and right here the real work is done. Ribosomes (microscopic protein factories) eagerly knot and tie together hundreds of thousands of amino acids (the smallest protein building blocks) in order to form a new hair shaft or to push out stronger hair shafts.

Secret No. 23

The rain, the cold, and even snow are your hair's best friends. Never forget that you're still in some ways a chimpanzee.

24 The Nutrients Your Hair Needs

Wherever we look around in nature, we can see that every creature and every plant has to be fed in order to stay alive and healthy. We realize that even microscopic-sized life forms have to be fed in order to stay alive and healthy when we put any cell of these animals or plants under a high-tech microscope. There are not many nutrients on earth which plants, animals, or human beings can consume. There are twenty different amino acids (protein building blocks), thirteen main vitamins with about one hundred different derivatives, probably thirty different trace elements like copper or iron (nobody yet knows exactly how many we need), seven minerals such as potassium or calcium, about a dozen of certain fatty acids like linoleic acid, glucose (the smallest building blocks from carbohydrates), and water.

Our hair needs all of those. Why? It is because our hair is not an isolated part of our body. It originates from our internal body, and despite being internal, the entire organism needs all these nutrients, every minute of every hour. Our hair-building cells crave their favorite nutrients. In the manner that bones prefer calcium and our eyes prefer vitamin A, our hair likes the vitamins B_2, B_6, and C and the trace element zinc—mostly to promote growth.

- B_2 is highly concentrated in milk and milk products such as cheese, in poultry, fish, grains, salad greens, and vegetables.
- Grains, bananas, soya and tofu products, walnuts, cashew nuts, liver, spinach, and avocados are rich in B_6.
- Fresh fruit or fresh-pressed fruit juices are the best suppliers of vitamin C.
- Large quantities of zinc are concentrated in oysters, liver, egg yolks, muscle meats, lobsters, snails, eels, and all kinds of grains like wheat, rye, barley, oat, millet, buckwheat, or spelt.

Many people, especially women, have a zinc problem, a significant zinc deficit that will hardly ever be recognized. They are very often almost void of zinc instead of having the zinc depots in all seventy trillion cells always completely filled. The reason for this is that large amounts of zinc are needed in glands like the pituitary or the suprarenal gland, which synthesize and secrete, with the help of the enzyme-donor zinc, important stress hormones. Stress hormones like ACTH, cortisol, glucagon, or epinephrine, to name just a few, help you to cope with all your stress factors during the day. So, the more you are under stress—at home, at your place of work, or wherever—the more zinc is released from your zinc depots.

That is why your hair lacks the important trace element necessary for growth. That is also why people with personal or professional problems often suffer from hair loss or from thin, brittle, and dull hair. The problem: Other than with B- or C-vitamin depots, it may take months to refill empty zinc depots in your cells. Good advice from modern scientists: Take zinc drugs (lozenges, for instance) for a period of thirty or even sixty days in order to get rid of your zinc deficiency. After two or three weeks you may realize that your hair (and also your nails) grows much faster.

Secret No. 24

Vitamins B_2, B_6, and C and the trace element zinc are your best companions for better hair growth.

25 Chase Off Free Radicals from Your Hair Cells

These free radicals actually aren't very hostile or malicious. Their job on earth is to kill everything that is weak or sick. They would never do any harm to molecules or cells which are protected, immune-protected, that is. So as long as your hair-building cells are well-protected, they will never be threatened by free radicals.

It is autumn and a lonely leaf spirals down from the branch of a tree. It finds its final resting place on the ground; one half yellow and brown, faded and dead; the other half still youthful green. When we stop by a few hours later, the entire leaf is faded. What happened? Free radicals—within a short time and obeying the order of nature—killed all the remaining living green plant cells.

Another example: You are invited to a party and it lasts into the early morning hours. It's four o'clock in the morning when you get home. It was fun, though—dancing, flirting, and talking, with all that noisy music, and everybody smoking (many of them smoking those big, thick, horrible cigars; it is modern, they say). You can cut the air with a knife and not more than a few hundred molecules of oxygen are left for sixty-two people in those rooms. Then add on the healthy offerings of potato chips and chocolates.

At home there is a stranger in the mirror. Some old person, perhaps five or eight years older than you are. The hair is brittle, thin, and lusterless. The face is also gray and without luster. The free radicals had taken their chance, gnawing at all your cells, particularly the ones in your hair. Sleep well and eat healthy food and within a few days, you will have regained the lost years.

By the way, there are four substances that offer almost all the protection for your hair. They include the antioxidants vitamin A, vitamin C, vitamin E, and the trace element selenium.

Secret No. 25

*Take antioxidants—
the mighty four—
from your pharmacy
for younger hair
in 30 days.*

26 Retain, or Even Restore, Your Natural Hair Color

Pigment molecules, similar to the ones in the iris of your eyes, have their little workshops within your hair cells. Day and night they work mixing up the same color, handing it over to the colleagues who do the rest of the work. As people become older, the pigment workers complain more and more that they aren't sufficiently supplied with raw material any more. All they can do is sit down and helplessly watch the hair shaft grow out of the body without pigments—in the gray or white color pure protein has.

Here are the reasons why your pigment workers are not getting enough raw materials any more:

– You are becoming older. The stomach produces too little gastric acid and the pancreas produces insufficient amounts of enzymes, so nutrition is not properly broken down anymore. Insufficient amounts of vitamins, trace elements, or other nutrients reach the hair cells.
– The immune system becomes weaker. Immune substances are withheld in the body and they cannot protect the hair cells and the pigment workshop any longer.
– Daily stress factors are not as easily dealt with as when someone is young, and stress devours nutrients.
– Very often elderly people have to revert to canned or microwave food because they are not mobile enough to purchase fresh, nutrient-rich foodstuffs on a daily basis.

Do you want to retain or get back your original hair color? Then supply your hair cells with the raw material they expect:

– The B vitamins, pantothenic acid (also called B_5), Para-aminobenzoic-acid (PABA), folic acid, and biotin build a family which works sufficiently in your intestines, as well as in the hair cell. Create your own "hair-color food" with foodstuffs rich in these vitamins such as liver; cold-water fish like trout, mackerel, halibut, cod, or salmon; all kinds of grains; all kinds of nuts and kernels; egg yolks; cheeses; soya and tofu products; and natural, unprocessed rice.

– Your hair pigment molecules are synthesized by tyrosine (an amino acid) with the help of the trace elements copper and zinc as enzyme donors. Do not worry about copper—your cells contain enough of it. Take zinc drugs for a period of thirty or sixty days. The interesting thing about the building block tyrosine is that it is a precursor of your happy makers and good-mood hormones, norepinephrine and dopamine. That is why faint heartedness or depressive moods and hair that gets gray or white too early often go hand in hand. Therefore, be sure to ingest more tyrosine by drinking the juice of one lemon or a little apple vinegar mixed with water before your main meals. That will give you more than enough tyrosine in your food, whatever you eat. The goal is to have all the protein nutrition in your food—like in your tasty barbecued steak—disassembled and sent from your intestines through the mucosa, via your blood, right into the pigment workshops of your hair.

Secret No. 26

Unbelievable, but true— you can change your hair if you eat properly.

27 Silky, Smooth, Fuller Hair— and No Dandruff: How to Wash Your Hair

Similar to your skin your hair has to "fight," or cope with the "hostile" outside world and at the same time protect your body. Your hair is like a mother who sacrifices herself for her children, fighting off whatever is not welcome—and very often she receives too little help for herself. It definitely is not an easy life for a hair cell to struggle against radicals, the cold, heat, rain, wind, and snow and at the same time work on pushing out that wonderful strong and healthy hair shaft, without even one single hour's vacation a year.

Our hair can be admirable. But instead of admiring it, some people hate their hair because it becomes old and gray and brittle, splitting all over with hundreds of hairs in the comb and dandruff on the shoulders. So instead of asking nature to "please, help me," they walk into beauty salons to purchase a pack of hair care products. Lotions, shampoos, tinctures, sprays, and strengtheners do little; they just torment the hair cells, never helping them.

The sebaceous glands of your hair react to your environment. It can be damaging for your hair and skin when, for instance, the rooms in which you work or live are too dry or overheated, when you wear hats that are too tight, or when there is smog or stinking clouds of exhaust gas. Your ancestors lived a natural physiological environment, clean and oxygen rich.

All that sebum your glands may pathologically over-produce (causing seborrhoa) will become rancid, mixed with dead, peeled-off protein particles. Your skin cells are not able to breathe any more and they degenerate into symptoms of an extreme over-proliferation. That is when dandruff sets in. It may be persistent because it is often not very easy to eliminate.

Don't torment your hair skin with any cosmetic products at all in case you do have problems with dandruff.

Buy a good medicinal shampoo at your local pharmacy. Water—nature's finest product—is the only other thing you need. Forget tight headgear; your hair hates it. Don't run away from every raindrop. Let your hair get wet, soaked with heaven's wonderful present. Your hair will love it. Take a hot/cold shower at home and dry your hair under your electric hairdryer.

You will not have to worry about dandruff or brittle and splitting hair anymore.

Secret No. 27

Do you have dandruff or brittle hair? Ask nature for help— not anyone else.

28 Your Hair Wants to Be Prehistoric—It Does Not Want to Be Pampered

True, our ancestors, hundreds of thousands of years ago, didn't know how to operate a PC. They never heard of Microsoft. They may have been stupid. But were they really?

I think not. They lived in harmony with nature. Anthropologists tell us that they played and laughed much more than we do.

Each and every one of their cells was healthy.

Our genes are amazing witnesses to their way of living. They haven't changed since. Our hair envies the hair of our ancestors. It took evolution millions, even billions of years, to produce the gorgeous mechanism of a single hair shaft. Our hair desperately yearns for that kind of environment—it doesn't care for high tech at all.

Give your hair back a little bit of that kind of physiological living—fresh air and plenty of physical exercise. It will do wonders for your hair as well as the rest of your body and mind.

Anthropologists tell us that people in those times had two or three hours a day of physical activity. That means they were running around hunting, digging out tubers and bulbs, collecting firewood, or just playing. The pores of their hair skin were wide open for absorbing oxygen. And even more of these life-giving molecules were swarming through the blood into their hair cells, bound to iron in the hemoglobin, the red blood pigments of the erythrocytes, the red blood corpuscles.

Oh, how each and every hair shaft loved that! In case one of these ancestors could join your barbecue party, your other guests would say: "It is rather difficult to have a talk with her about Jasper Johns, the Met, or even the new features of the new BMW. But her hair, I have to admit, is the most brilliant I've ever seen in my life."

Learn from those people, your ancestors. Do as much exercise in fresh air as you can, even if you can't afford hours of walking or jogging over the trails close to your home. Twenty minutes, ten minutes, even a few minutes will do. These precious minutes will be a personal present to your hair, giving them at least the feeling again of what they were genetically designed to do. Hair cells can be so happy, so extremely joyful.

Secret No. 28

The fantastic duo— oxygen and physical exercise. Make your hair proud again.

29 Brittle Nails—Why?

About 90 percent of people with brittle nails lack gastric acid. Nails are up to 99 percent keratin (as is your hair and your epidermis, the outer skin layer), and keratin is nothing other than a certain compound of protein.

We have more than enough protein in our food. There is more than enough in hamburgers and steaks as well as in vegetable food. The problem is that protein in our nutrition has to be dissolved and disassembled. It is done first by gastric acid. Drink the juice of one grapefruit or lemon or a little apple vinegar (dissolved in water or apple juice) before your main meals—and your metabolism will enjoy a massive influx of amino acids (protein building blocks) into keratinocytes (the nail-building cells).

The intake of pancreatin drugs (from the pharmacy) for a period of thirty days may help you even more. They contain dissolving enzymes—lipase for fat, amylase for carbohydrates and protease for protein—everything that your pancreas normally secretes into the digestive juice of your small intestine. The nutrition pap in your intestine can no longer be completely dissolved if your pancreas is weakened. A weakened pancreas can develop when your diet consists primarily of sweets and processed foodstuffs.

Try it out. You may be surprised to realize that the odor of your stool has been neutralized within just twenty hours. That means that all the fats, proteins, and carbohydrates in your food have been broken down and their tiniest parts—fatty acids, amino acids, and glucose— are fortunately on their way to your seventy trillion body cells to keep them well nourished and healthy.

You will also realize that your nails will regain a smooth consistency in just a few days.

Secret No. 29

A well-tuned digestive system keeps brittle nails away.

30 What Your Nails Need

You may paint your nails red (or cinnabar, purple, or black), but that will not make them healthier.

Unattractive white lines or points and taming often appear. These are symptoms of a zinc deficiency, which can be relieved with the intake of zinc lozenges. Grooves may be symptoms of a protein deficiency. Drink lemon or grapefruit juice or apple vinegar (mixed with water) before every main meal. A deficiency of vitamin A may be the reason for nails to split. Vitamin A-rich foodstuffs include all yellow, green, or red fruits or vegetables like apricots, berries, melons, pumpkin, paprika, carrots, spinach, broccoli, and chard. When fingernails are too flat, an iron deficiency may be the reason. It can be a sign of too little protein when they are brittle, or when they break or splinter easily

Indications of constant (day and night) mental or physical stress are first revealed on the fingernails. Even the nightly stress while you are sleeping—grief, sorrow, affliction, trouble—damages your nails. Unsightly nails are also a symptom of overexertion.

A 38-year-old secretary with two kids, gets up in the morning at 6 A.M., showers, gets dressed in a hurry, fixes breakfast for her husband and the kids, shouts good-bye to her little daughter on her way to the school bus, takes her boy to the kindergarten, works all day, eats lousy food at the canteen, does the shopping, cleans the house, picks up the kids from volleyball and the guitar lessons, takes care of everything else, and finally staggers into bed at 11 P.M. How can this poor exhausted woman ever find the time to maintain and properly care for her nails?

Secret No. 30

Follow the previous advice and attempt to reduce stress.

Enjoy Better Hair and Nails Within 30 Days

- *The follicles are the sources of beautiful hair—
so feed them properly.*

- *Your hair wants to protect you—not vice versa.
Allow it to be exposed to the rain, the snow, and the cold.*

- *B vitamins and trace elements are responsible for hair growth.
Choose the right foodstuffs.*

- *Protect your hair from free radicals.
This allows you to attain a more youthful appearance.*

- *Yes, it is true—you can eat color into your hair.
Eat foods which contain necessary pigment molecules.*

- *Wash your hair with the correct shampoo. Remember that the shampoo you choose determines to a large degree the condition and appearance of your hair.*

- *Your hair needs oxygen and physical exercise.
Learn from your ancestors.*

- *Brittle nails often occur as a result of a poor diet.
It will take you just 24 hours to solve that problem.*

- *How are nails effected by stress? Try to cope better with stress and you will notice a marked improvement.*

THE PERFECT 30-DAY PROGRAM FOR STRONG BONES AND TEETH

31 Bones Often Complain— and We Don't Listen to Them

Bones can't talk, but if they could, they would reveal the truth about careless treatment and foolish indifference. People care about their external appearance and neglect what is inside.

Our bones are a very specialized kind of connective tissue, evolutionarily developed as creatures grew larger and expanded their territorial domain. Human bones consist of the compact outer bones and the rather sponge-like inner bones with the bone marrow. The inner bones offer the marrow the best possible protection, and that is really necessary as it produces all of our red and white blood cells.

There are three different kinds of bone cells which cooperate fabulously: 1) the osteoblasts, which build up the bones, 2) the osteocytes, completed bone cells already implanted into the bone structure, and 3) osteoclasts, large cells that are able to absorb bone mass. Our bones consist mainly of the minerals calcium and phosphorus, though a good chemist can trace out hundreds of other substances.

Our bones have the highest calcium turnover of all our tissues. That means that they need large amounts of fresh calcium as a result of releasing expended calcium. According to the calcium we ship to them and also according to the burden we allow them (in addition to other factors), our bones are never—not even for a minute—at exactly the same condition. They become weaker and stronger at different intervals and to different degrees all day long.

Secret No. 31

All you have to do to develop powerful bones is to support the strengthening and reduce the weakening phases.

32 Swallowing Calcium Tablets Is the Worst Thing You Can Do

Maintain a healthy nutrition and physical exercise program and you will retain perfect bones throughout your life.

Of major importance is the mineral calcium. Every adult is the proud owner of approximately 1.2 kilo of calcium—men more, women less, of course. Ninety-nine percent of that mineral is part of the bones. The remaining one percent plays a vital role in the nervous system. The organism devours that essential mineral out of the calcium reservoir found in the bones whenever the concentration in the blood is too low.

This is just one of the reasons why people, particularly those under nervous stress, have weak bones and perhaps loose teeth.

Swallowing calcium tablets is the worst thing you can do. The vital bone minerals, calcium and phosphorus (and also magnesium), always have to stay in a physiologically healthy relation in order to build up the hydroxyapatite in your skeleton, a concrete-like crystal grating. Scientists speak of the optimal calcium-phosphorus ratio.

Too much calcium or phosphorus can damage your skeleton. Not more than one-tenth of it will be absorbed from the intestine into the blood, sometimes not even 4 or 6 percent when you swallow tablet calcium (like calcium gluconate or calcium carbonate).

That is the least of your problems. Calcium, in the form of a mono-preparation, removes phosphorus out of the body via the kidneys and bladder. (By the way, psychiatrists and neurologists sometimes give their patients calcium tablets in order to reduce pathological over-concentrations of phosphorus.) Taking calcium tablets decreases phosphorus absorption in the intestine from the normal 70 percent to a critical 30 percent or even less. It depends on the number of calcium tablets one takes. To maintain a physiological ratio in the blood again, phosphorus will be drawn out of the bones, which makes them weaker. Taking more than two to four grams of tablet calcium daily also means there is a risk of insufficient iron utilization and also of kidney disease.

Even worse than too much calcium in the blood is over-absorption of phosphorus. Almost all industrial processed foodstuff or instant meals like pizza, hamburgers, sausage or meat meals, are extremely high in phosphate—the phosphorus-salts. The same holds true with soft drinks like cola or lemonade. Swallowing a hot dog with a can of cola is a pure phosphate bomb.

What happens after that? Seventy minutes later certain glands are alerted. These glands now pump plenty of hormones into the blood. The parat-hormone steals the skeleton's precious calcium in order to maintain a healthy calcium-phosphorus ratio again. It really is a vicious circle.

Secret No. 32

Eat cheese and maintain the desired calcium and phoshorus ratio.

33 The Nutrients Your Skeleton Needs

Calcium is the most important nutrient your skeleton needs. Supply your bones with this mineral in a healthy ratio with other substances like phosphorus. That way you won't confuse your organism, your intestines, the kidneys, blood, or bones causing them to eliminate this or that nutrient to stabilize the physiological balance. All kinds of cheeses, milk, curds, yogurt, almonds, nuts, figs, egg yolks, legumes, cabbage, spinach, fennel, fish, and chocolate are very rich in natural calcium.

There are many people, particularly women, who claim that they eat plenty of cheese and have weak bones in spite of it. That can be true, as nutritional calcium is dependent on gastric acid (similar to protein and iron) in order to become solubilized. This means being ionized, or electrically charged. The mineral can take part in the manifold actions of your metabolism just by being ionized. Otherwise unsolubilized calcium will be deposited in your joints, causing arthritis, or even under your skin, causing wrinkles. Drink a spoonful of apple vinegar, mixed with water, before your main meals. That is the way you can ensure that you create more gastric acid.

You have enough phosphorus or phosphate, respectively, in your daily food. Try to cut down by avoiding hamburgers, pizza, or sweet drinks.

Your bones also contain plenty of magnesium. Why not take pumpkin seeds, almonds, cashews, peanuts, hazelnuts, walnuts, or sunflower for a little in-between-meals snack? All are magnesium rich.

Nature deposits large amounts of vitamin B_{12} into your bone-building cells. These cells are connected to a miles-long labyrinth of wafer-thin blood vessels from where the vitamin slides over to the bone cell. Here it participates in the development of new bone mass. Liver, kidney, meat, and fish contain much vitamin B_{12}. Vegetarians can satisfy their B_{12}-household requirements by eating sauerkraut or yogurt. The fermentation in these foodstuffs will produce vitamin B_{12} molecules.

Vitamin K (in cabbage, spinach, broccoli, salad greens, green beans, cucumber, and cauliflower) participates in the joint operation of calcium and vitamin D, but never forget that your skeleton needs healthy nutrition with all kinds of vitamins, minerals, and amino acids every day, not just the few mentioned here.

Secret No. 33

Perfect food makes you stronger—and for a longer period of time.

34 How the Sun Can Determine the Strength of Your Bones

The sun is not only a warming fireball for our body. The sun controls and rules us. Nature invented the vitamin D molecules, because the photons, these tiny parts of the sunbeams, have no physical power. They are the messengers of the sun and are synthesized in cholesterol-containing skin cells which transport the power of this mighty celestial body right into the nuclei of all of our seventy-trillion body cells. They stimulate genes to crank up the cell metabolism as transcription factors.

Besides that, vitamin D has more important jobs to do. Vitamin D helps the mineral calcium by passing through the mucosa of the intestine into the blood and installing calcium salts into bones and teeth. Furthermore, vitamin D regulates our phosphate balance and also the calcium-phosphorus ratio, a crucial mechanism for a healthy skeleton. Vitamin D is fat soluble. It is absorbed in the intestines with the help of bile, transported as 25-hydroxycalciferol to the kidneys. There it is dynamically charged and ready to cooperate in the development of bones.

Vitamin D, which is metaphorically nothing else than the sun itself, gives your bones their power. That is why it is crucial to expose the skin to bright light. The older you become, the more sunlight your bones need. You can help your skeleton additionally by eating D-rich foods—cold-water fish like mackerel, salmon, halibut, tuna, codfish, trout, and sardines in oil. The same holds true with liver, kidney, milk, eggs, and grains. Cod-liver oil is an excellent vitamin D-rich supplement, but don't take it, teaspoon-wise, longer than a week, as fat-soluble vitamins can accumulate to toxic concentrations in your tissues.

Secret No. 34

The sun works efficiently. A walk of just 50 minutes in the bright sun strengthens your bones.

35 Osteoporosis Is a Bone Problem Afflicting Mostly Women

During and after menopause, women increasingly lose the ability to synthesize estrogen. This hormone prevents the deterioration of bone mass and also cranks up the calcium uptake of the skeleton. Estrogen also increases the production of another hormone, calcitonin, which ensures that there is not too much calcium withdrawn from the skeleton.

What makes it all worse is that after their last menstruation, women often lose enormous amounts of calcium in the morning, excreting the precious bone substance with the urine. Under "normal" conditions, by nourishing themselves the "civilized" way with junk and microwave food, they will never be able to balance this fatal loss. This is the reason why women after menopause often lose up to one and a half percent of their bone mass every year.

This syndrome is called osteoporosis. It can lead to broken knuckles if the person moves the wrong way.

Women after menopause synthesize less vitamin D in their skin, another factor contributing to this disastrous illness. Moreover, they lose the ability to transform vitamin D into the biologically active form calciferol. Besides that, they eliminate too much proline, a protein building block, which is part of the raw material of collagen and bone mass.

Here is the good news—you can easily stop the fatal progress of osteoporosis.

1) Vitamin C (in fresh fruit) activates the input of calcium into the skeleton.
2) The trace element boron (in vegetables, nuts, and fruits) prevents the pathological excretion of calcium with the urine.

3) Eat or drink calcium-rich foodstuffs like cheese, curd, yogurt, or milk.
4) Let the bright sunlight caress your skin, at least once a day for twenty minutes.
5) Activate the function of your suprarenal gland. It may partially compensate the decreased production of estrogen. Give her the cholesterol-rich raw material she needs like grains, seeds, and lecithin as a supplement.
6) Commit yourself to a physical exercise regime.

Secret No. 35

Fight off osteoporosis. Help your bones, and nature will help you.

36 Put Stress on Your Bones—They'll Like It

An interesting thing is our genetic adaptation to our environment and lifestyle. Our genotype, the sum of our 80,000 active genes, remains the same, guaranteeing each one of us the characteristics of a human being. Others, the phenotype, determine the manner genes transcript and form the individual characteristics of humans; one individual is red haired, the other one brown haired; one is short, the other one tall. Their phenotypes are different—but they are all human beings.

The phenotype can be influenced. This means that the phenotype adapts to whatever internal and external determinants exist. Inherited hair color, geographical location, and physical exertion are just a few of the internal and external determinants. Moving from Chicago to Miami will stimulate pigment-producing genes that give you a darker suntan. Doing sit-ups or knee bends will stimulate genes, thus allowing muscles to develop. Your phenotype changes in such cases.

What is the upshot? Everybody's phenotype is influenced according to how he or she lives, nourishes himself or herself, adapts to a different climate, and so on.

Your skeleton is also malleable. The extent to which you put stress on your skeleton determines its strength. This is the reason why bones never—not even for one minute—stay the same. The strength of your bones depends on your diet and the degree of stress you place on them. They are very sensitive to all kinds of changes and adapt accordingly. You are stimulated by genes, which have the job to adapt your body to changes in your environment, your way of living, and so on. This is one of the most important acquisitions of nature during trillions of years of evolution. This is the way creatures (and even plants) stay viable within changing environments.

If that were not so, many genuses would have become extinct. Sixty-five million years ago the dinosaurs became extinct, probably because a huge meteor hit the earth, leading to violent climatic changes on earth. It was impossible for the giant animals to genetically adapt to these environmental changes in such a short time.

Nevertheless, you have enough time to genetically strengthen your bones by just adapting them to more stress and better nutrition. Continue reading to find out more about how to give your bones more power in the following chapter.

Secret No. 36

Exercise your bones— and your genes will do the rest.

37 Strengthen Your Skeleton with Weights

Every step you take increases the gravity placed on your skeleton. When someone is sick and confined to bed, there is almost no pressure on his or her bones, and the skeleton becomes weak. The first step out of bed accelerates the recovery rate of the skeleton. Nourishing your skeleton well is just half of what you can do for strong bones. Work out with weights and do other types of exercise, and all your bone cells will be reinvigorated and generate youthful bone metabolism.

They really look nice, these blue, red, or yellow (or even pink or mint) two-pound weights you see displayed in your sporting goods store. You can tie them around your calves, over the ankles, hold them in your hands, or tie them around your wrists. They increase the gravity and the pressure on your skeleton. That way you can—at least in the beginning—shorten the time of your workouts. The efficacy of a three-minute training program with four 1-kilo weights (around wrists and calves) is equivalent to almost thirty minutes of exercise without these weights.

Exercising with the weights for the first time will rejuvenate your entire skeleton. Within just three minutes—it is unbelievable! Researchers claim that people would do it a couple of times every day and sometimes would not stop at all, if they knew how beneficial a workout like that is to their skeleton. Physical activity, especially practiced with small weights, decreases the susceptibility of bones to fracture and diminishes the risk of osteoporosis or bone loss.

Prevent injury by warming up before exercising. One or two minutes of stretching will help you avoid injury and improve your performance. Warming up increases the flow of blood, nourishes your bones (and your muscles), and raises your body temperature. Muscles and bones will be more flexible and that reduces the risk of an injury (please read more about physical exercise and fitness in the following chapters of this book).

Any kind of exercise will do your skeleton good: aerobics, jazz dance, walking, jogging, cycling, mountaineering, swimming, or tennis. Commit yourself to never using an escalator or elevator when going up. It is also highly advised to use a trampoline. Jumping (you can do that on a small home trampoline) increases the gravity on your bones while exercising. It also stimulates the cell metabolism more efficiently than walking or jogging.

Secret No. 37

Let your bones experience the reason they were created.

38 How to Rejuvenate Your Joints

Do your joints hurt? Do they prevent you, at least sometimes, from doing exercise and sports because they are somehow immovable and stiff?

Joints are flexible connections between your bones, attached with strong, but elastic, bands of connective tissue. Their joint caverns are cushioned with cartilage, so the bones will not rub against each other and cause ailments, discomfort, or pain. Additionally, joints work like the shock absorbers in your car. They are filled with synovial fluid, a jelly-like lubricant. Cartilage and synovial fluid contain high concentrations of proteoglycans, substances which can—like a sponge—absorb plenty of water and mineral salts. The proteoglycans enable your joints to glide like a greased piston.

Our poor joints are extremely strained. When the helpful proteoglycans thin out (because of bad nutrition, for instance), the joints may very quickly dry out and lose their mobility. This is the way it develops most of the time. The synovial membrane, which tightens the fluid in the joint capsule, swells and this is followed by the exit of joint fluid. The cartilage becomes weakened, rubs off, inflammations supervene, and the first pains come along. Warning symptoms in the form of pains will particularly arise when the joint is undercooled and at the same time strained.

Joint problems are always conditioned by poor nutrition, except as an aftereffect of a traumatic action, such as an injury. The joint cells are badly nourished over perhaps many, many years. Cartilage, synovial fluid, and proteoglycans are weakened; free radicals attack the defenseless cells; the influx of immune substances like white blood cells, prostaglandins, or leukotrienes leads to inflammations—and the cycle continues. Fever-causing pyrogens and mediators like cytokines worsen the symptoms, nerve fibers are overstrained, and tissue hormones stimulate the disassembly of cartilage or also of muscle mass. You consult your doctor, and he utters the dreaded word—arthritis.

Make sure that you eat properly. Your joints are highly dependent on nutrient-rich foods. Moreover, try not to expose your joints to cold or wet, as long as they are not warmed up by sufficient blood flow. If you suffer from arthritis, wear woolen joint-warmers during sleep for the first one or two weeks. Dress warmly. Showers should not be too cold. Always consider that having joint problems means that the joints have undergone faster aging than the rest of the body. So, give your joints their youthful years back. It is not at all difficult.

Secret No. 38

Your joints are sensitive. They may need more attention and care than other parts of your body.

39) Teeth: Gain Admiration and Influence People with Those Pearly Whites

You have thirty-two of these remarkable little white creatures. Teeth have a hard job everywhere in nature. They have to tear apart all kinds of food, sometimes rather tough foods like stale old bread or stringy meat. The funny thing is that teeth love to do that hard job.

The alveolar bone, the strong jawbone, has the highest calcium turnover of all tissues in your body. Another superlative? The enamel, which covers your teeth with a fine layer, is the firmest substance in your body.

Archaeologists are always surprised that thousands-of-years-old skeletons show wonderfully healthy teeth. "This person is 4,200 years old and has better teeth than I, and I am not more than forty-four," they would say. Modern nutritionists know that bad teeth are caused by bad food and that's all there is to it.

Similar to bones, teeth primarily consist of calcium and phosphorus. Looking at the enamel or the white tooth substance, you would say that there are no blood vessels at all. What a mistake! The microscope uncovers a fascinating world. The enamel itself may be as hard and polished as titanium on a space shuttle. In spite of that, there are infinitely numerous tiny channels and tunnels, through which atoms, or tiny molecules, or just ions, which are charged parts of atoms, can slip through onto the surface of your teeth. Beneath is the dentine, where channels and tunnels become larger as they are on alert to transport vitamins, minerals, and proteins. Your teeth want to be supplied with nutrients from the inside and want to be protected by immune substances in your blood and by immune substances in your saliva.

The Cavity Dilemma and What You Can Do to Avoid It

Nobody wants to have cavities—and your teeth do not want to have them either.

Do you know what a cavity is? Precisely stated, it is tooth decay. It is an open invitation to all kinds of bacteria to immigrate into the oral cavity, enthusiastically shouting, "Oh, it's great here! Fantastic place, a paradise! It's warm, wet, and there is plenty of sugar coming in every one or two hours."

Eating and drinking food with sugar and processed grain (like spaghetti and bagels) fills the oral cavity with nutrition pap. Food particles remain after breakfast, lunch, or dinner unless removed by cleaning the teeth and that does not happen too often so there are these residues. They attract bacteria wherever remaining food particles are within our digestive system.

The trouble with bacteria (and with viruses, fungi, parasites, and other microbes) is that the more you feed them, the less moderate or easily satisfied they are. It's a strategic error and also a fallacy or a false conclusion to negotiate with the chief of 1,000,000,000,000,000,000,000 bacteria by telling him, "Okay, we give you one more caramel candy, but then you guys have to leave the oral cavity—all of you, understand?"

They never will leave because they are malicious. The chief would say "Forget about that caramel candy. I heard him ordering pizza with sweet soda. Therefore, we will get enough stuff to eat." Bacteria are capable of producing another 1,000,000,000,000,000,000,000 grandchildren and so on. Fortunately, a bacteria generation does not last twenty-five years like that of humans, but just a few hours or even minutes, if we are lucky.

When you eat a chocolate bar, the bacteria in your mouth eat the sugars, digest them, and leave organic acids that attack the enamel. That does not take any longer than ten minutes from the moment you swallowed the sweet. The remainders, produced by bacteria, make the saliva and the film on your teeth acidic.

The bacteria attack on the enamel intensifies should someone continue to eat sugar. Whenever he or she stops eating or drinking sweet things, bacteria will find no further nutrition and will no longer attack the teeth.

Tooth decay is the most chronically spread infection. Bacteria that induces cavities are called streptococcus. Most people, even doctors, refer to them as streps. When the oral cavity is free of streps, you may eat as much candy, chocolate, and sweets as you like and you will never, ever be in risk of developing cavities.

On the other hand, streps reproduce by the trillions in your mouth within a very short time—the moment you swallow pizza with cola. Sucrose, besides glucose the smallest carbohydrate building block, belongs to the favorite dish of bacteria. It creates glucanes out of it, a polysaccharide, which attaches to the surface of the teeth as kind of an organic tissue layer. This insoluble, sticky, and adhesive layer will at the same time offer shelter for thousands of colonies of streps.

Bacteria's Paradise

- *Bacteria find the homes they look for within the tiny, sticky, caverns of the plaque layer.*

- *Like marmots or bears before their hibernation, they provide for the future, synthesizing fructane out of sucrose, the sugar. This specific polysaccharide is storable, so bacteria—which are very clever—can re-synthesize it to edible carbohydrates again.*

- *That way, of course, a permanently acid milieu develops and damages the teeth. Nibbling sweets in the late evening in bed is the worst thing you can do.*

- *Sweet fruits also contain sugar that can be used by bacteria. Sweet apples, bananas, or grapes (also raisins) contain up to 15 percent sugar while oranges, peaches, or berries can contain up to 8 percent. The same holds true with sweet fruit juices, even if they are self-squeezed.*

- *Plaque bacteria metabolize carbohydrate components and form organic acids, which stick as a gelatinous mass of gram-positive bacteria, saliva proteins, lipids, and undigested polysaccharides to the surfaces of the teeth.*

- *Fermentation of that mass starts minutes after a sweet or carbohydrate-rich meal or snack and may continue for hours. Synthesized acids cause the pH to fall into critical regions between 5.3 and 5.7, when enamel demineralization takes place.*

- *Eating sweet snacks or drinking sweet liquids (sugar-sweetened coffee, for instance) keeps the pH in your oral cavity permanently (all day long) in the critical regions. That means permanent acid attacks on the enamel, inevitably leading to tooth decay.*

- *Bacteria like it!*

Cheese, particularly ripe cheese, is a perfect natural "drug" against tooth bacteria. For example, you eat a highly sweetened fruit salad out of the can—and while you are still eating, the pH in your saliva and mouth falls to a pathologic pH of, let's say, 5. Take two bites of cheese afterwards and your pH will immediately rise to a harmless 7. The high content of proteins, calcium, and phosphorus neutralizes the plaque acids. Cheese also stimulates the reconstruction of teeth.

An important protection substance of your teeth is the saliva, as long as it is not sweet or acidic. Women, after menopause, sometimes suffer from a lack of saliva production. This often leads to dry oral cavities. In such cases the bacteria are not washed or rinsed out properly by swallowing sufficient amounts of saliva. Besides, saliva is rich in certain immune substances such as immunoglobulins, which kill bacteria.

Fluorides, like in fluoridated tablets, liquids, salt, or toothpaste, will protect teeth and prevent cavities. Clean your teeth thoroughly after every sweet or carbohydrate-rich meal or snack. A sugar-free chewing gum will help produce more saliva. It will also press cleaning and protecting saliva into the microscopic crevices in your teeth. You should also brush food particles out of your mouth. White points are the first warning symptoms of a demineralization of your teeth enamel. Stop eating sweets and start taking care of your teeth.

Secret No. 39

Help your teeth to fight off bacteria—today!

40 Strong Gums for Health and Beauty

Firm and strong gums provide for optimal digestion and they make anybody look young—making their smiles and laughter attractive. So, why not do all you can to maintain healthy gums?

It is often just a matter of vitamin C. The first warning symptom of vitamin C deficiency is the reddening of papillar bodies, the slight skin elevations between the teeth. It may be the beginning of gingivitis (inflammation of the gums) and periodontitis or periodontal disease (when the entire attachment apparatus of teeth to the alveolar bone in the jaw is weak or sick).

Bacterial plaque is the major pathologic evil-doer, though there may be other factors. The gums become inflamed if they lack vitamin C. They will swell, the gums become loose, and they will start to bleed. Tiny capillary vessels will tear, and bacteria and other pathogenic microbes can intrude into the vessels, the cells, and the tissues. Besides, free radicals take their chance to ultimately destroy the protecting membranes around gum cells. They will also destroy the cells themselves. The gums shrink, the teeth stand out naked and ugly, slowly become loose, and eventually fall out.

Plants also have capillary vessels. They protect themselves with their own vitamin C, which is one of the reasons why they produce this essential nutrient. The finer the blood vessels are, the more vulnerable they are. Therefore, your gum capillaries also urgently need protection. Do your gums bleed after biting into an apple? Try it first when eating that apple. The more fresh vitamin C-rich fruit you eat, the more your gums will be protected and healthy.

The ligamentous attachment of your teeth to the jawbone wants to demonstrate how powerful it is, so chew stringy foodstuffs such as stale bread. Chewing a sugarless gum will also help, by strengthening your attachment apparatus and massaging your gums.

Secret No. 40

Vitamin C is your gums' best friend.

You Can Develop Strong Bones and Youthful Teeth and Gums in Just 30 Days

- *Eat calcium-rich food—your skeleton needs the precious mineral.*
- *Do not take calcium tablets. They will upset the fine balance between your calcium, phosphorus, and other nutrients.*
- *Fuel as much vitamin D from the sun as you are able.*
- *Commit yourself to regular physical exercise.*
- *Get yourself little weights for your daily work-outs.*
- *Put stress on your bones—climb staircases.*
- *Protect your joints with good, natural food and keep them warm.*
- *Fight the bacteria in your oral cavity—for beautiful teeth.*
- *Take in more vitamin C—your gums need it.*

LOSE WEIGHT THE NATURAL WAY IN ONE MONTH

41 Forget About All the Diet Quackery and Empty Promises

Probably the simplest mechanism in our body is that of storing and losing fat. Mother Nature wants us all slim because only creatures that are not overweight can survive and pass on strong genetics to upcoming generations. Nature does not like to see people running around with a couple of extra pounds. You would never see this with animals or plants. The only exceptions are pregnant mother animals or those who prepare (like grizzlies) for the long, cold, winter months without fine honey.

The mechanism of lipogenesis (storing up fat) and lipolysis (releasing fat out of the adipocytes, the fat cells) is simple. Storage fat (triglycerides) is exclusively used for burning as a fuel. Whenever you are under stress, your body has to react with concentration, alertness, physical response, or whatever. That means that the metabolism of seventy-trillion body cells has to be cranked up, fired up by burning fuel. In addition, there are just two kinds of fuel around in your body, glucose (the smallest building block of carbohydrates) and fat. Take your pocket calculator and figure it out. There are seventy-trillion cells and each one of them burns, let's say, twenty or fifteen, okay, just ten triglycerides a second—oh, God, okay, make it ten a minute. That adds up to seventy-quadrillion fat molecules being burned in the time you need to check out the night's TV schedule.

Being overweight often means being unattractive, an attribute that most people would like to change. So people or companies often promise you a plan to lose weight with products or programs, which "aren't too expensive." Sometimes it looks as if everybody wants to make money from those who are overweight by promising them a miracle.

These unfortunate men and women have fat as a barrier to living better, feeling better, being thought of in a better light, and gaining greater status and approval. They also lessen their chances when looking for a job or a partner by being overweight. It is always those five, ten, or more pounds that block them from their legitimate goals. Listen to girls around the corner table of the cafeteria, "Burt is after me, but he is too fat"—even if Burt is just three pounds overweight. The company boss tells the personnel manager, "Whenever you employ somebody, take a slender one, male or female. Our company is famous for hiring the slender, slim, and dynamic ones, while the competition pays the bill for the fat, lazy, and inactive ones. It's what we call corporate identity."

That is why you read so much about easy ways to weight loss. There is a lot of money involved. Do not trust them. Trust nature, your very best friend. Nature shows you how to get rid of your excess fat.

Secret No. 41

Whatever you do or plan to do—trust nature first.

42 How Do People Get Fat?

Let us say there are two newborn babies—two girls. Both have the same amount of fat cells. Both have the same amount of pre-adipocytes, empty cells with just a ridiculous content of 0.01 micrograms of fat each. These, by the way, are the kind of fat cells Canadian and Alaskan bears store up in October in order to survive the winter.

The two mothers are happy. From time to time, they get together with other moms. "I haven't got any problem with my little kid," the one mother says. "Whenever she cries or is unruly, she gets the bottle with a sweet solution. That makes her calm and she looks so blissful. No problems at all."

What this mother probably does not know is that the more sweets the baby drinks, the more the baby's liver will transform it into triglycerides, the storage fat. Glucose, the smallest building molecule of carbohydrates, and fat are both made out of just three elements: oxygen, carbon, and hydrogen. In addition, the liver is adept in converting pizza or bagels into belly fat. The more carbohydrate it converts into fat, the more pre-adipocytes will be filled up and converted into real fat cells.

These two girls are now thirteen. Both are slim like young birch trees, everybody insisting neither of these two will ever become overweight. However, one of these two slender girls already has two-and-a-half times more fat cells than the other one. Ten years later, the young women are at the blossoming age of twenty-three. One of them is fourteen pounds overweight and the other girl still is slender.

The problem is that once there is a fat cell, or a pre-adipocyte being converted into an active fat cell, it can increase in size almost indefinitely. The fat cell absorbs ugly brown and yellow fat, growing and growing—200, 300 times and more the original size.

People become fat because nature wants to help them. That is the nature of their cell's metabolism. Eating pizza with cola and ice cream, candies, and cakes fills the intestine with easily soluble carbohydrates like sugars and the real fat. The liver converts it all to storage fat, the triglycerides, because nature has the impression that the person is a bear out of honey, and winter is approaching, so he has to store as much fat as he can in order to survive the uncomfortable and dreary months in that cave under the big oak tree.

Secret No. 42

People become fat because their liver converts fat out of sweet and easily soluble carbohydrates.

43 The Worst Thing You Can Do Is to Eat Fat, Sugar-laden Foodstuffs, and White Flour Products Together

Your Christmas turkey with all the trimmings will never make you fat or even overweight. You can even enjoy a thick porterhouse with French fries. However, never drink something sweet along with it or have a sweet dessert immediately afterwards. You ordered venison with yellow boletus and rice? Go ahead and enjoy your meal, but do not order that tiramisu or that fine sweet French liqueur the waiter told you goes well with your meal.

The moment you eat white flour or unprocessed rice or eat or drink something sweet, hormone-like particles in your saliva recognize it by chewing and tell the great news, via hormonal signals which are faster than lightning, to certain enzymes within the soft crossings of blood vessels, extracellular fluid, and fat cells. These enzymes (scientists name them lipoprotein lipase) are now alert and await all those delicious fat molecules in order to shuttle them into the fat cells.

As you can easily see, the fateful one-way street can be created just by chewing a plain bagel. The street of fat goes from your mouth to the stomach, to the intestines, crossing the intestinal mucosa into the blood, to the liver, and farther via the blood stream right into the insatiable adipocytes (the fat cells in your belly, the buttocks, and the thighs).

Drinking sweet soda and eating anything sweet will catalyze the condition, making it even worse. In addition, never forget that anything sweet combined with fat (to include the hidden lipids in your hamburger or hot dog or the "open" fat in your ham) leads to an uncontrolled influx of fat particles into your fat deposits.

Start by just skipping the sugar-loaded drinks. That will make it a lot easier for you to lose weight. The one-way fat street into your adipocytes will be blocked and your fat cells will open and release triglycerides to be burned as fuel in your seventy trillion body cells.

Secret No. 43

Hot dogs and ice cream are the best fat makers you can imagine.

44. Growth Hormone Has Been Nature's Most Important Fat-Burner for Hundreds of Millions of Years

Why not imitate free-living animals or our kids? Lose weight while sleeping. That is how nature has arranged it by storing this genetic program into each one of us. Here is how it works.

The home of this genetic weight control program is your pituitary gland. It is about the size of a cherry pit, and it produces eight hormones. Hypothetically, if you could squeeze this little gland between your thumb and forefinger almost nothing but water and growth hormone would spurt out. The other seven hormones are concentrated in extremely negligible amounts. This proves how important Mother Nature considers her wonderful growth hormone.

Around seventy minutes after we fall asleep at night, the pituitary gland becomes very busy. It synthesizes enormous amounts of growth hormone, blood concentrations increasing up to forty fold or even higher within a very short time. The little growth hormone molecules all have tiny golden keys. They swarm through all 60,000 miles of blood vessels in our body, at first opening adipocytes (fat cells) and releasing their contents, the yellow triglycerides, and our storage fat. Growth hormone is a stress hormone. Only stress hormones have the ability to open fat cells, which are very often locked and barricaded like Fort Knox.

These triglycerides are transported via the labyrinthical blood streams to all seventy trillion body cells in order to be burned to energy. Growth hormone is also active in these seventy trillion body cells, not only in the fat cells. The hormone molecules repair and rejuvenate the cells, which are often very badly damaged during the day's stress. We owe it to the growth hormone (and, of course to other substances like enzymes or proteins) that we most often look younger in the morning than in the evening. Free-living animals and our kids owe it to that hormone to wake up in the morning slender and full of energy.

So why don't overweight persons lose weight while sleeping? These people very often wake up not only with unloved extra pounds, but they are tired. The answer is simple: their pituitary gland produces an insufficient amount of growth hormone. In some cases—pathologists know that by dissecting deceased patients—the gland of 50- to 60-year-old people ceases to synthesize any growth hormone.

Moreover, why doesn't the gland produce any slimming and rejuvenating growth hormone? There is also an answer.

The Miraculous Growth Hormone

❇ *In order to synthesize just one of trillions of growth hormone molecules during the night, the pituitary gland has to put together 191 amino acids, the smallest protein building blocks.*

❇ *This means that the hormone molecule is rather bulky. In addition, the poor little gland (well, not poor, actually, she really likes the job!) exerts maximum performance during hours.*

❇ *Nevertheless, without the raw material of sufficient amino acids, the pituitary gland may just synthesize a meager percentage of growth hormone molecules of what she really is supposed to produce. Instead of 100 percent (to make you slim and look young), just 80, 70, 56, 42, or just 22 percent is produced. There is no chance then to unlock fat cells or to do all that rejuvenating maintenance in seventy trillion cells while sleeping.*

❇ *Putting 191 amino acids together—and doing that trillions of times during night—the gland needs helpers. The most important helper is vitamin C which is used as an activator or enzyme donor. This is the reason why the little pituitary gland has the highest vitamin C concentrations of all tissues in your body.*

❇ *In the early morning when it is still dark outside, the pituitary gland is not exhausted at all, having undergone that tremendous effort. Now it slowly stops the growth hormone machine. It then activates the awakening mechanism and activates the day's hormones.*

The best advice for more growth hormone: Right before going to bed in the evening, eat a snack of "pure protein," about one ounce of fish, cold meat, or chicken (without the skin—chicken skin is the worst cholesterol bomb), vegetarians can substitute with tofu. Drink fresh-pressed lemon juice. Eat nothing else—no bread, no toast, nor mayonnaise.

The lemon juice will help create gastric acid, so the protein will be sufficiently digested during the first hours of sleep. A steady influx of amino acids will pass the mucosa of your intestines and reach all of your cells—a necessary precondition for the recovering of weak cells. Furthermore, your pituitary gland will happily greet the arrival of trillions and quintillions of amino acids. With the help of the vitamin C in your lemon juice, the gland will synthesize growth hormone molecules, always netting together 191 amino acids at a time and secreting the molecules into the bloodstream.

Growth hormone is the great nightly slim-maker. It activates your metabolism to burn off the triglycerides in your buttocks, thighs, or belly. Besides, you will turn back your biological clock and maybe regain lost years. In addition, when you wake up in the morning, you may feel mentally better, more optimistic, and more cheerful. For the first time in a long time, you will hum a song in the shower.

Secret No. 44

A little meat, and a little lemon juice before going to bed, and your fat tissues will not have a happy night.

45 Other Perfect Fat-Burners: Sun, Iodine, and Fruit

Probably the most mysterious molecule in our body is a releaser hormone synthesized in our hypothalamus (another gland in our diencephalon the innerbrain) thyrotrophin-releasing hormone (TRH). What actually makes it so mysterious is it is also one of the tiniest proteins in our body. TRH consists of only three amino acids. Other proteins consist of thousands of these protein building blocks.

TRH is the germ of life in our body. The molecule wanders about an inch distance to the nearby pituitary gland and activates this gland to secrete another hormone, thyrotrophin (TSH), the substance which stimulates the thyroid gland to synthesize and secrete her thyroid hormones into the blood.

These hormones are similar to agents of the yet unknown "workshop of life" in our body. Nobody, including researchers and scientists, so far know how life comes into being. Nevertheless, they know the mechanisms of the thyroid hormone molecules. They hustle around through the labyrinth of blood vessels and visit all of our seventy trillion cells. There they light matches (metaphorically speaking) and inflame the mitochondria, microscopical tiny burning chambers, where fat or glucose are burned to cell energy.

Cells, that do not receive visits from these thyroid molecules, will die. Cells, which are only visited by a few of these molecules, will burn just a little fat or glucose. When there is a rush of these thyroid hormone molecules, cells will burn plenty of fat or glucose. In other words, people with sufficiently working thyroid glands produce plenty of these little fat burners.

A thyroid hormone (There are several different ones.) consists of two parts iodine and one part tyrosine (an amino acid). Many people live with a permanent iodine deficiency, and may have permanent problems with their fat tissues. All they would have to do is substitute their regular kitchen salt with iodized salt or sea salt.

People living on or close to coastal areas always have iodine molecules on their tongue (brought by the wind from the sea). This is one of the reasons why they do not accumulate fat as easily as do other people.

Because the thyroid hormone molecules also are rather small, they are easily attacked and destroyed in the bloodstream by free radicals. Without the help of immune police, many of these precious molecules will not reach their destinations—the cells. Vitamin C is their best ally. The more fresh fruit you eat, the more your sensitive thyroid hormone molecules make their way to the mitochondria of your cells. That is why people living in "fruit countries" do not as easily become fat as people living in areas where the freshest fruits are five-week-old radiated strawberries in the supermarket.

The sun is also very helpful in reducing weight because it stimulates the activity and slimness genes, which help to increase the cell metabolism. That means that more energy is necessary and more fat fuel has to be burned. Allow your body the bright daylight or sunlight as often as possible in order to take advantage of this process.

Secret No. 45

Slim down the tropical way.

46 Calorie-Reduced Diets Tend to Make One Fatter, Not Slimmer

When someone reduces his or her calorie intake—let us say from 2,000 daily down to only 1,200—an interactive hormone signal compound wakes up, "We're getting too little food, so we will have to maintain our reservoirs." Then comes the order to the fat tissues to lock their depots and possibly to not give any triglycerides away anymore. Our organism and the metabolism are not dumb. They still carry the genetic experience of millions of years of evolution. In addition, they own a tremendous genetic memory. "Looks as if there is a famine coming up," they would say. "We human genes had plenty of those in our long history. I tell you, be stingy with your nutrients as much as you can, and retain fat. This famine coming up may hold on for months or even years."

Therefore, the iron bars on the fat cells lock and the padlocks click into place. No depot fat to be burned anymore.

However, this person stays alive and is under stress, and, of course, needs plenty of energy fuel. So, where does one receive this fuel? The first source is the fast-burning glucose, 300 grams of glycogen-reserve is in the liver, blood, and muscles of a woman. Men have a little more, about 400 grams—just enough to take care for three or four hours energy supply of nerve and brain cells when someone is under stress. These cells only accept glucose as fuel, no fat, because the brain and nerves have to be as fast as lightning when danger arises, when prey has to be caught. The fat-burning process would take too long.

Therefore, this particular person undergoing a starvation cure burns his or her glucose within a short time. Glycogen depots empty, no fat available. So what to do? One possibility would be to take that word starvation literally.

However, such is not the case. In cases like that Mother Nature has taken precautions because otherwise many, many of their amazing creatures would die out just because there is no more glucose or fat, which would mean no fuel at all to burn for life-giving cell energy. So nature—during evolution—made about fourteen of the twenty amino acids that are glucoplastic. That means the liver (and the kidneys) can transform body protein into glucose. Scientists call this process gluconeogenesis.

So our Mr. or Mrs. Dietmaker will first lose about 400 grams of glucose and approximately 1,500 to 2,000 grams of weight as there are three molecules of water attached to every glucose molecule. This is the first sign of "success" of every calorie-reduced diet.

The organism next devours protein out of the entire body in order to fulfil the needs of gluconeogenesis or energy gaining, respectively. In addition, as our connective tissue participates with 25 percent of our entire protein depots, much of that wonderful collagen will be sucked out, broken down into amino acids, a part of which then are transformed into burnable glucose.

It is in this manner that the person loses his or her beauty, youth, complexion, and health—in other words, losing everything but real fat. As soon as the diet is over, the fat cells will be greedily hoarding new triglycerides, increasing the fat tissues on thighs, belly, buttocks, or hips.

Secret No. 46

Do not put your faith in starvation diets.

47 A One-Way Street Named Fat

Like everyone else, our body also loves habits. We do certain things always in the same manner—how great! Happily adapting to circumstances or environment, our body would call it. A few examples: Our organism loves the same time span of sleep, the same wake-up time in the morning, and walking with the dog every early evening on the same path day after day—up to the fork in the road, turning left, into the trees, down the east lakeside, and then home again. Even the dog loves that routine.

Our body likes being slender and staying slender. Nevertheless, it can change its mind sometimes loving being overweight and remaining overweight. The body would just change perhaps one of thousands of genetic codes which control its weight. That would be no problem—genetic researchers call that mutation.

Responsiblity for being hefty is very often due to point mutations, when only one single position in a gene is affected—and genes have up to hundreds of thousands or even millions of such positions. Those point mutations may occur when someone smokes too much or is living isolated, with no friends or love. Perhaps he moves from Tucson, Arizona, to Nome, Alaska. There are thousands and thousands of possible point mutations, and many of them, or even most of them are adapting the concerned person to certain habits—like eating too little, too much, or physiologically wrong.

Then the one-way-street fat may be established from the intestine via mucosa and blood to the liver, from there directly into the fat tissue in the belly, thighs, buttocks, and hips. People whose fat metabolism is forced into that one-way street may even starve by eating nothing, merely living on chewing gum and coffee. They may never lose weight because night and day, there is a steady stream of triglycerides from the intestines into the adipocytes, the fat cells, like the Mississippi River which wouldn't carry any water at all or would rather dry out than flow backwards.

The following chapter informs you how to turn the one-way-street fat around, so fat molecules would really stream out of the fat cells, being burned by seventy trillion cells.

Secret No. 47

Why people don't become slim—the one-way-street fat is genetically encoded.

48 Insulin: The Fat Tyrant

The crucial role to building up the one-way-street fat is insulin, a hormone of the pancreas. Insulin is—so to say—the best friend of billions of fat cells, like a night watchman who controls the padlocks on all fat cells being locked as prescribed. As long as there are elevated insulin concentrations in the blood, the adipocytes keep and hold their content.

Insulin is the hormone that transports glucose (blood sugar) into the cells. Whenever glucose molecules pass the mucosa walls into the blood stream, the pancreas also excretes a corresponding amount of insulin molecules. Insulin keeps your blood-sugar level healthy. However, as long as the glucose molecules are not yet transported from blood into the cells, the insulin concentrations will remain increased. In addition, as long as they remain increased, the fat cells would not surrender their triglycerides. This is because insulin is an anabolic hormone, storing fuel like glucose and fat, and promoting fatty acid synthesis. This means, that as long as the insulin concentrations are elevated, the fat cells are waiting for further fat shipment and are not at all prepared or even willing to give fat away. This is how the one-way-street fat is established.

Therein lies the problem of a high percentage of all overweight people. When they remain overweight for a long time (many months or years), their genes will consider that a habitual situation. In order to adapt that being, they would initiate one or a few point mutations. This will cause corresponding changes in proteins for which these genes are responsible.

One consequence may be a syndrome which scientists call insulin resistance and which makes many people overweight. Cells have insulin receptors on their membrane. Fat cells, for instance, have up to 250,000 of these landing spots, because they need the hormone for synthesis of triglycerides. The problem is that the more glucose you have in your blood (because you may just have swallowed a grandiose cup of ice cream), the more insulin your pancreas secretes. Simultaneously the cells cut down the amount of their insulin receptors in order to protect themselves from too much triglyceride fat at a time.

Scientists call this phenomenon the down regulation. It increases the fateful overconcentration of insulin. Sometime the affected person will develop chronically elevated insulin concentrations, making no difference how much she or he does or does not eat. She or he will never lose fat.

That is the one-way street of fat.

The dilemma of many people who deprive themselves of food almost to the point of starvation is that they never become slim.

Escape that one-way street by just skipping white-flour products (like noodles or bagels) and anything sweet, including sweet drinks. There will be less insulin excreted from the pancreas into the blood and cells will increase their insulin receptors again. Automatically, the cells can easily swallow whatever insulin is concentrated in the blood. Blood insulin goes down, and the one-way-street fat turns around, just like a bridge with one lane that opens for traffic from either side, controlled by signal lights. Green would mean the fat stream flows out of the fat cells into the burning chambers of all body cells.

Secret No. 48

Omit white-flour products and anything sweet and avoid the fatal fat traffic.

49) How Does Physical Activity Help in the Removal of Fat Cells?

Thanks to modern scientists—now at the beginning of the new millennium! They supply us with so many new discoveries. Actually, they have done nothing else than unravel nature's fascinating puzzles. Well, thanks anyway.

It is all very easy, in fact. Muscle cells, for instance, burn the most fat. The highest percentage of fat is transformed into energy by the heart muscle cells, because the heart is the most powerful muscle in our body. The volume of protein synthesis determines the power of a cell, which takes place in molecular-tiny protein factories called ribosomes. The more ribosomes a muscle cell contains, the more fat it will burn.

The heart cell of a healthy person possesses roughly 200,000 ribosomes, which tie together amino acids to essential cell proteins. In addition, such a cell owns about 1,000 mitochondria (tiny ovens that burn fat) producing cell energy. The more physical activity we undergo, the more ribosomes and mitochondria our muscle cells have and the more fat they will burn.

Our kids romp about all day giving their muscle cells numerous big and luscious fat burners. The same is true with free-living animals. Just hanging around all day and doing very little, decreases ribosomes and mitochondria drastically—down to possibly just 20 percent of the original quantity. So cells, particularly muscle cells, can burn just 20 percent fat of what they physiologically would be able to burn.

The good news is that the quantity of ribosomes and mitochondria change from minute to minute. When you sluggishly drag your feet out of your house with not more than a miserly 32,000 ribosomes and 170 mitochondria in each of your muscle cells, then do twenty minutes of sharp walking or jogging—you will return to your home with possibly three times as many of such tiny fat burners. So, help your body slim down with physical exercise.

Secret No. 49

Boost your cell metabolism and lose even more fat with exercise.

50 What to Eat, What to Avoid

Thanks to all the computer and high-tech innovations, our brave and competent researchers now use analyzing machines to enable them to watch cell processes in the femto-molregion, what would correspond with one quadrillionth part of a gram (a quadrillion is a one with fifteen zeros, by the way). To put it in a more understandable way, they now watch the bustling, city-like life in every cell like through a show window.

That way they can gaze at that fat metabolism in wonder. "Uh-huh, that's the way it is," they may say by surprise. It now becomes evident that there are lipolytic (fat-burning) foodstuffs and lipogenic (fat-incorporating) foodstuffs. All an overweight person would have to do is eat the "lytics" and skip the "genics."

What to Eat

- Fruit
- Vegetables, legumes
- Salad
- Uncooked vegetarian food
- Mushrooms
- Whole meal, full-grained products
- Soya or tofu products
- Natural rice
- Potatoes
- Milk and milk products
- Eggs
- Skinless poultry
- Lean meat
- Fish

What to Skip

- Sugar, anything sweet (like chocolate), sweet drinks
- White-flour products
- White rice
- French fries
- Sausage
- Fatty ham or bacon
- Fatty meat
- Poultry skin
- Mayonnaise, dips, dressings, or sauces
- Cakes, pies, cremes, puddings, pastries, cookies
- Ice cream

Slim Down with Genetic Help in 30 Days

- ❋ *Don't trust any diet promises.*
- ❋ *Never consume sweet and fat foodstuffs and white-flour products together.*
- ❋ *Melt fat with your growth hormone by snacking on a little meat or fish plus lemon juice before going to bed.*
- ❋ *Believe in the "Amazing Three:" iodine, sun, and fruit.*
- ❋ *Calorie-reduced starvation cures tend to make one fatter, not slimmer.*
- ❋ *Reverse the one-way street named fat to "burning."*
- ❋ *Solve your insulin problem—in case you should have one.*
- ❋ *Boost burning fat with physical exercise.*
- ❋ *Eat the right foodstuffs, and eliminate the wrong foodstuffs.*

Secret No. 50

Eat the "lytics," skip the "genics."

PSYCHE AND NERVES: HOW TO BECOME A HAPPIER PERSON IN ONE MONTH

51 Your Genetic Happiness Code

Free-living animals like titmice, gorillas, or even voles fall asleep within two seconds and wake up in the morning within a split second. They enthusiastically enter the new day, focused and euphoric. They have to because the moment they move, they already are in danger of being attacked by a predaceous animal.

Nerves and brains of free-living animals are controlled by an interactive system of genes, hormones, and neuropeptides, which makes them aggressive and "optimistic" as long as they are awake. These animals do not experience violent mood swings between bliss and despair. That is, of course, because they do not have a consciousness like we human beings have.

If, hypothetically speaking, a golden eagle had a consciousness, he would never experience pessimism, hopelessness, or anxiety like we often do. This is because his brain and nerve cells are well fed, and running at 100 percent metabolism. That is the way nature wants it. The brain and nerve cells of all creatures are well fed, arming them for competition and rivalry, for the struggle that is endless.

Each one of us still maintains the genetic code of optimism and euphoria because of our genotype. The sum of all our genes has hardly changed since the days of our ancestors, the chimpanzees. Our genotype coincides with the genotype of chimpanzees by 99 percent. Significant differences are just consciousness, frame, and skin. Comparing cells of a chimpanzee and a human being would hardly show any difference.

All we have to do is feed our brain and nerve cells well and—what is as important—allow them the necessary recovery, by resting and sleeping.

Secret No. 51

Every one of us can wake up blissful, happy genes.

52 What Makes People Uneasy, Fearful, and Even Desperate

Nature is like a kind-hearted mother to us. When our brain and nerve cells are undernourished, they place a feeling of dejection, melancholy, or even anxiety over us as a benevolent protecting precaution. Nature does not want us to run into risks or to accept challenges for which our organism is not sufficiently prepared.

That is how nature also handles it with all her free-living animals. When a rabbit escapes a fox, it will flee into the shelter under a hedgerow. While trembling and shaking, the rabbit's brain and nerve cells are robbed of all nutrients under the tremendous stress of being chased. It will take a while until the rabbit's cells will have substituted the extreme loss and deficiency of proteins, vitamins, or trace elements. Not until then does the animal dare to leave the shelter.

It is the same with us. Being timid, pessimistic, or when we avoid conflict situations signals biochemical deficits in our brain and nervous system. Mother Nature wants to take us by her hand and lead us into a shelter (a peaceful, silent room, for instance), consoling us, saying, "Rest, my dear. Your brain and nerve cells are so pitifully looted. I do not want you to be harmed. Do not take any risks now. You are sick, my dear."

Every one of us has experienced the puzzling change of moods. You wake up in the morning, cheerfully saying, "This will be a great, happy day," then three hours later, you are so inexplicably discouraged. Where do these mood changes come from? Mother Nature makes you competitive for stress situations, kindly filling your brain and nerve cells with anxiety. Always depending on how well or badly your brain and nerves are nourished, your metabolism levels may reach 100 percent, 90, 75, 48 percent, or less.

Consisting of seventy trillion cells, our organisms function in a rather complicated way. However, the way Mother Nature leads us through life is very simple. Becoming slim is simpler than we believe. Falling asleep is simpler than we think. Becoming a happier person is also easier than we think. Read more about that in the following chapters.

Secret No. 52

Being timid we feel the kindness and love of nature. She now surrenders her most affectionate mystery— how happiness grows.

53 Feed Your Brain and Make Your Nerves Happy

Your muscles like to burn fat for energy. Your brain and nerve cells strictly burn glucose, the tiny building blocks of carbohydrates, because glucose burns more easily. Brain and nerves have to make quick decisions, so they need a fuel that gives them a lot of cell energy within a split second. Burning fat in a cell is like setting a briquette on fire. Burning glucose is like holding a match to the butane of your gas cooker. That is, incidentally, the reason why nature has structured the glucose molecule so simply. It can rush out of the intestine into the blood and particularly into the brain and nerve cells.

Supplying these cells with glucose is the first step on your way to becoming a happier person. Glucose is also referred to as blood sugar. So as long as the blood-sugar concentrations are within a physiologically healthy range, your brain and nervous system merrily burn glucose and are as energetic as a young sparrow. If the level is too low, the cells are undernourished, making them as energetic as—let's say—an old crocodile. This leads to a syndrome called hypoglycemia. You will be tired, even chronically fatigued, nervous, and restless. These are the first warning symptoms.

A normal blood-sugar level is somewhere between 80 and 120 milligrams per 100 milliliter of blood. Diabetics who produce too little insulin (which transports blood sugar into cells) can reach levels of 300 milligrams or even higher. If the level goes far below 80, like down to 65 or even 55, it often stimulates craving for something sweet. Because the glucose in sugar is released quickly, it promptly increases the blood sugar level, which makes the affected person feel better. Women are more often affected than men, because they have smaller glucose reservoirs, called glycogen depots. Hypoglycemia is one of the important risk factors for being overweight.

The problem is that the quickly-soluble glucose gets the alarm bells on in the pancreas that now secretes plenty of insulin into the blood. In addition, this hormone makes the blood-sugar level fall—mostly down to an even lower point than before. The brain and nerve cells run out of their fuel glucose again—and the craving starts up again—a vicious circle.

It gets even worse when the level dips—often rapidly—down to a low point of 45, 40, or even lower. People open the liquor bottle because alcohol also rushes into the blood in form of glucose, and within seconds into the brain. The hypoglycemic candidate feels wonderful—for a very short time. Then the level rapidly goes down, and the craving for alcohol pushes him to open the bottle again.

Feeding your brain and nerves to happiness means definitely skipping anything sweet.

Substitute all white-flour products (like bagels, toast, or bread) for full-grain products. They contain complex carbohydrates, which will be broken down in your intestines in a slow process, dispatching glucose molecules into the blood over several hours. Therefore, the blood-sugar level can remain high, though brain and nerve cells are continually sucking their glucose fuel out of the blood.

The breakfast should be enriched in protein with fewer carbohydrates. Foodstuffs your brain and nerve cells prefer include cottage cheese, tofu, meager cold meat, roast beef, chicken meat (without the skin), fish, shrimp, and pumpernickel and wholemeal bread. Try, for instance, shrimp cocktail with pineapple or other exotic fruits, mayonnaise (lowfat), and a few slices of wholemeal toast. In addition, drink coffee, tea, or whatever you prefer—without sugar, of course. You will be perhaps surprised how much better you feel throughout the entire morning, without that typical loss of vigor and phases of fatigue and without the craving for sweets and chocolate.

Your brain and nerve cells are filled with their fuel—which is the first important step on your way to feeling better and happier.

Secret No. 53

Allow your brain and nerves to reach their energy fuel—and they will reward you with more vigor.

54 Step Number Two: Relax Your Nerve Cells

Bad nerves are very often the cause of misfortune, lack of success, or even the cause of tragedies when, for instance, a couple gets divorced just because they both lose their nerves, either one labeling the other as being self-centered, always been self-centered, and never have been anything but an egocentric. Okay, that is a reason for getting divorced (their lawyers would say), however, nature does not find that appealing. Nature does not like to see couples (even animal couples) separate because of bad nerves.

Having bad nerves may mean failing the application interview, finding no partner for life, or not even having friends. Bad nerves mean shortcomings and inadequacies.

Biochemically, bad nerves mean something entirely different. There is a myelin sheath around every brain or nerve cell, which is thick and oily and wrapped around the cell in fleshy layers to protect the cell. Sometimes sheaths of more than 100 layers may be wrapped around a nerve axon like a rather endless rolled-up rug. That illustrates how important it is for nature to see our nerves well protected. Myelin is an electric insulator, essential for the signaling of nerve impulses.

These myelin sheaths have a certain viscosity—not too dry and not too wet. If they were to dry out, you would have the feeling of "exposed" nerves, and be always irritated, restless, or nervous. The condition of these sheaths changes from day to day, hour to hour, depending on how much stress you have to fight and what you ate at your recent meal. When someone says that he just does not find inner rest and peace anymore, that could mean bad nerves or damaged myelin sheaths.

Three recently-discovered major genes generate the permanent forming of new relaxing myelin. Now there is the dilemma of many stressed and hyper-nervous people. Their myelin sheaths thin out because of stress and junk food. The nerve cells beg the genes emphatically to get the production of protecting the myelin going. But the genes must answer "Sorry. There are not sufficient nutrients in the cell to build up new myelin."

That is one of the reasons why many people have very bad nerves.

Myelin consists predominantly of cholesterol, proteins, and sphingomyelins that are compounds of fatty acids, phosphates, and choline, a vitamin that is considered to belong to the B family. Choline is of enormous importance for keeping cholesterol in liquid state. Without choline the myelin sheaths will lose their viscosity, and will "glue" the nerve cell membranes—nervousness will be the inevitable consequence.

Without choline, cholesterol will become rancid (not only in the nerve cell membranes, but within the entire organism) and will mix with dead and scaling proteins, further plastering over the myelin sheaths. Nervous signaling will be slowed down; thoughts are just tormenting themselves from nerve cell to nerve cell. The affected person is not only irritated and nervous, but also unable to concentrate. Even worse, the electrical potential of the cell decreases. Nutrients will be not sufficiently transported into the cell. The connection between hormones and neurotransmitters, which transmit nervous stimuli, will be disturbed. Emotional deficits may arise as well as frigidity, coldness, and emotional deprivation.

This is all because nerve cells and their axons and the nodes of Ranvier are not wrapped physiologically with myelin.

Go to your pharmacy or drugstore and get yourself natural lecithin, which contains up to 40 percent choline. Mother Nature offers you a gift to make your nerves healthy. It may take just thirty-six hours to you calm down. What great new layers will wrap around your myelin sheaths! Soon, you may say you feel great, that your nerves are calm. You may feel prepared for stress and conflict situations.

Secret No. 54

*Choline may—
if you're lucky—
free you from
nerve problems.*

55 Happiness Rises Out of Tiny Nerve-cell Vesicles

In our restless, hectic world, we meet so many people who lament, "I don't know what is wrong with me. A few years ago I was delighted by little things like a flower, a falling star, and a tiny bug curiously glancing up at the stem of a daisy. How do I feel now? There is nothing I can enjoy. I cannot get enthusiastic nor can I fall in love. I feel like an empty bottle."

Happiness is made in metabolic workshops, the same way a closet would be manufactured in a carpenter's workshop. The carpenter uses wood as material, our brain and nerve cells use tyrosine as their raw material; The more tyrosine someone has stored in the tiny vesicles of his brain and nerve cells, the more happiness he or she can produce out of this material.

Tyrosine is an amino acid, a protein building block. It is synthesized within neurons by another amino acid (phenylalanine) or is absorbed from the extracellular fluid, where all of our cells are bedded. In a few steps of biosynthetic pathways, the neuron workshops change the tyrosine molecule to dopamine and then to norepinephrine. Both are called neurotransmitters. They transmit our good moods throughout our organism and body.

The "Happy-Makers" Within You

❊ *Dopamine is the substance which gives us well-balanced moods, a steady and inner serenity, and a blissful mental peace. It produces the happiness of older people. The older we get, the less dopamine we convert to norepinephrine, the impetuous neurotransmitter creating a euphoric state.*

❊ *Norepinephrine is the "happy-maker" of young people and of those in midlife. Nature has invented it in order to put creatures into sort of a positive aggressive condition whenever they depend on it by chasing prey, by being chased, by watching and controlling the environment for beasts of prey—and for reproduction, searching for the right partner, fighting competition off, producing charisma, and putting on a grandiose seducing show.*

❊ *What makes norepinephrine also so precious is another occurrence. This neurotransmitter takes care of opioid peptides like the endorphins, uplifting drugs we synthesize within our own metabolism. Norepinephrine elongates the half-life period of these narcotics, so the more norepinephrine we have stored, the more slowly opioid peptides will be metabolized. We are then able to maintain enthusiasm, happiness, and blissful optimism.*

When all the trillions of delighting dopamine and norepinephrine molecules are manufactured, they will be stored in synaptic vesicles, which means within the gap between two nerve cells. Now whenever the kids come merrily running home from school, shouting "Mommy! Mommy!," Mommy's synaptic vesicles open, and trillions of neurotransmitters sparkle criss-cross throughout her nervous system and brain, producing a hot and sweet flood of blissfulness.

For a long time the pharmaceutical industry has tried to imitate nature or make it even better. It is hopeless. They failed to copy a norepinephrine or dopamine drug, which brings happiness from a bottle of capsules into our body. Therefore, they tried it another way —to develop a drug which stops the metabolization of these fantastic neurotransmitters. They label these drugs monoamine oxidase inhibitors. There are plenty of those on the market, prescribed by neurologists or psychiatrists.

The newest triumph of the pharmaceutical industry are re-uptake inhibitors. These drugs ensure that neurotransmitters will not be sucked out of the synaptic vesicles back into the watery cytosol of the brain or nerve cell where they are unable to transmit happiness. Both ways of artificially synthesizing good moods are against nature's intentions. Nature would grow re-uptake inhibitors and monoamine oxidase inhibitors on trees or bushes if it were so.

Crank Up Your Own Production of Happy Transmitters

- *It is most important to give your brain and nerve cells more tyrosine by introducing acid into your gastric juice before your main meals with lemon juice or apple vinegar (dissolved in water). The protein in your nutrition will then be better broken down.*

- *Soya-lecithin (available in health shops) contains up to 40 percent phosphatidylcholine. This vitamin occupies cholinergic neurons on the mighty vagus nerve. This nerve streaks through your digestion tract. The neurons—in case they hold enough choline—start firing the moment you spot the delicate foie gras on your dish. This will also stimulate secretion of gastric acid.*

- *A large amount of vitamin C is necessary for the metabolic pathways from tyrosine to blissful dopamine or norepinephrine, so allow your nerves and brain as much fresh fruit as you can. Many people are unhappy or even depressed because they lack this vivacious vitamin.*

❋ *Calcium is one of nature's best calming drugs and is necessary for transmitter release. Enrich your daily menu with milk, cheese, yogurt, or curd.*

❋ *If you take all this to heart, you may stimulate a chronic increase in electrical activity in your brain and nerve cells. That will stimulate the synthesis of dopamine- and norepinephrine-producing enzymes. Your nerve terminals will deposit more raw material protein, and the transmitter activity—sparkling happiness all over your nervous system—will be maintained over hours, not just minutes. You may feel newly born!*

Secret No. 55

Help nature produce the tiny "happy-makers" within you.

56 Meditating Like the Animals

There is one thing we can and should definitely learn from animals. They are highly focused and tremendously active as long as they are under stress. They do a 100 percent job, scientists would say. On the other hand, they are completely at rest as long as they are not under stress.

It is as if they had a switch to turn completely from action to rest and vice versa—like we turn the lights on and off with a switch.

Biochemically they switch within the vegetative nervous system from the sympathicus to the parasympathicus and vice versa. The sympathetic nervous system increases heartbeat, circulation, pulse, brain waves, and thyroid function—all what makes us alert. It decreases digestion and libido, which are not very useful during the competition struggle. The parasympathetic nervous system does exactly the opposite; it increases digestion and decreases activity. The total switch between both is crucial for the vital force of all free-living animals.

It may be crucial also for us to maintain a better switch. We are often not entirely "engaged" when we are under stress, because there are often too many stressful hours during a long day. It is even worse when we rest; the switch from sympathicus to parasympathicus is insufficient. We lay on the sofa for an hour or so, but still much too concentrated on the day's duties, or on our sorrows and fears.

It is not easy to cut them off. Nevertheless, here is what we can do to take care of an almost complete switch into a sufficient and recovering resting phase.

Go out in the nature or in a park on your own and remain for half an hour, entirely absorbed in yourself.
- Listen to the murmur of a brook.
- Watch the clouds float by.
- Watch the treetops swaying in the wind.
- Look at a green meadow.

When you get home, you will feel relaxed—and invigorated with your nerves calmed down, and your energy level increased.

Secret No. 56

Get back to the crucial switch in your vegetative nervous system.

57 In the Paradise of Sleep

There is a sleep hormone, melatonin, produced in your little pineal gland. You need it when you go to bed in the evening.

As with other important nerve substances, melatonin's precursor is just one amino acid, tryptophan. Nature does not want to make a big metabolic fuss to induce animals and humans to sleep every night. Sleeping and dreaming are too important.

Tryptophan is in your daily food, as are the other amino acids. When it has reached your brain via the blood stream, it will be converted into the neurotransmitter serotonin. Serotonin will then be transformed in the pineal gland to melatonin. All three substances are like triplets. It is not a problem at all for your metabolism to make the sleep hormone out of a simple food particle. That again demonstrates how important nature considers sleep for recovery.

Of the twenty different amino acids and particularly of all eight essential protein building blocks (which we absolutely have to take in with our daily nutrition), tryptophan is the smallest and weakest and in fact, is also the rarest one. One or two hours after a meal, all the absorbed amino acids swarm into the blood and reach the brain. Here are very narrow accesses, the blood-brain barrier. The crowding and pushing is rather ruthless. In addition, the weakest ones lose. Such is the case with tryptophan. The pineal gland waits in vain for her precious precursor.

Five thousand years ago Chinese doctors advised their emperors to sweeten their tea with sugar in order to fall asleep. This advice is still valid. Eating or drinking something sweet late at night provokes glucose and an insulin influx into the blood. Insulin will immediately transport not only glucose into body cells, but also the strong and heavy amino acids. That way the little tryptophan molecules will have less competition at the blood-brain barrier. There will be more tryptophan in the brain, more serotonin, and finally more of the sleep hormone melatonin.

Warm milk, sweetened with honey, may be helpful (or even one tablespoon of sugar though sugar is, apart from that, not at all recommended). Eat your dinner earlier. It should be not rich in protein (less meat, poultry, or fish), because digesting protein keeps your metabolism and your body and maybe your mind awake. A lot better for people with sleeping problems is a carbohydrate-rich dinner; for instance, spaghetti, for instance, with a well-seasoned, spicy Mediterranean tomato sauce.

Secret No. 57

Something sweet will let you dream.

58 How to Become a Winner

Being a winner or a loser is often just a fraction of a molecule away. It is this fraction of a molecule (the methyl group) that is the difference between epinephrine and norepinephrine. Both are stress hormones. They create a high level of alertness and concentration. They allow you to be more prepared to cope with all kinds of stress. However, epinephrine lacks the euphoric component that norepinephrine possesses.

Therefore, you may recognize which individuals are winner- or loser-types when they are confronted with stressful situations. The winners love stress. It makes them feel triumphant, active, and productive. The losers hate stress. It makes them feel inadequate. Epinephrine types tend to have a defensive reaction in stress; they avoid conflict situations. Actually, they avoid almost everything that requires physical or mental exertion.

Epinephrine is mainly synthesized in the adrenal medulla and transported via the bloodstream, what takes the molecules up to eight seconds to traverse the entire circulation. Norepinephrine is produced in postganglionic neurons of the autonomous nervous system. This "winner" molecule stimulates the sympathetic nerves, which are active in all "flight-or-fight" responses. Norepinephrine is transmitted faster than lightning within the nervous system, almost as fast as light particles themselves.

Nature's favorite molecule is norepinephrine, because it is more powerful, making creatures superior. Norepinephrine makes us euphoric and creative and stimulates our fantasy. When Mozart composed a divertimento, or Shakespeare wrote his plays, or when a two-year-old girl full of enthusiasm creates her first painting with mother's lipstick, or when Mom, also full of enthusiasm, plans the summer's vacation—they are all norepinephrine types. The losers, though they have one methyl group more in their molecules, lack all that fantasy, creativity, and euphoria.

The precursor of norepinephrine is the amino acid tyrosine (please read more about that in secret number 55). When brain or nerve cells are exhausted of tyrosine or when they were never supplied with this raw material, the adrenal medulla takes care of all the mastering of stress by providing plenty of epinephrine, because nature does not want to lose creatures because of a lack of tyrosine. Very often epinephrine acts as a substitution substance. It makes us at least viable—even without the winner-transmitter norepinephrine.

How do you fill your nerve and brain cells with victory power? Read more about that under secret number 55.

Secret No. 58

Become a winner by just giving away one ridiculous methyl group (chemically: CH_3).

59 How About Emulating Einstein?

"Fantasy is more important than knowledge" is what Einstein said, so cultivate fantasy in your kids. Well, he had it easy. He had plenty of intellect. No problem for Einstein to concentrate on more than five or six telephone numbers at a time.

The intellectual capacity of our brain depends on one important neurotransmitter—acetylcholine (ACh). Metaphorically speaking, it allows you to remember all the birthdays of 122 relatives and good friends. This neurotransmitter is synthesized in the cholinergic nerve terminals. One single enzyme does all the work as long as there is enough of the raw material choline in the adjacent extracellular fluid. Nerve terminals crave the B-vitamin choline, which is accumulated within brain neurons. The more ACh that is synthesized within these neurons, the greater the amount that will be released into the synapses of this neurotransmitter, and the more cholinergic neurons will fire rapidly—all leading to nothing less than perfect intellect.

The older people become, the more they lack the ability of synthesizing ACh because cholinergic neurons become necrotic and die because they are not sufficiently supplied with choline, the raw material of ACh. The first warning symptoms are forgetfulness and bad concentration; both typical symptoms of old age. Later dementia may develop to include Alzheimer's disease, which is a disorder of the cortical cholinergic system of the brain—determined by a decrease of ACh.

For better or even Einstein-like concentration, eat choline-rich foods: liver, soya or tofu products, egg yolks, walnuts, peanuts, almonds, mushrooms, natural rice, full-grain products, spinach, shrimp, and cottage cheese. The best nutrition supplement is soya-lecithin (available in health stores) which contains up to 40 percent choline.

Secret No. 59

You may never win the Nobel Prize, but you can make your brain a lot younger with more choline.

60 Bright Light and the Copper Enemy in Your Brain

We may feel terrific after experiencing the first prolonged sunny day of the year. We are suntanned, and we look younger and more attractive. In addition, we feel better because our mind has been effected. The trace element copper synthesizes the pigments in our tanned skin. In other words, there is now more copper in your skin. In addition, less copper is in your brain cells from where the tanning had drawn it out. Copper in the skin means an attractive complexion; too much copper in the brain can lead to nervousness.

Metabolism often uses two substances as antagonists. Examples include sodium and potassium, and zinc and copper. Either have to be in a physiologically healthy ratio or balance, respectively. Because zinc deficiency is one of the most common nutrient deficiencies (it shares this characteristic with folic acid deficiency, by the way), many people have elevated copper concentrations. This occurs particularly within their brain cells, the favorite home of this trace element. That is what causes restlessness, irritation, and other psychobiological symptoms.

Responsible for these symptoms are copper containing enzymes, which may be harmful throughout the body. They are necessary for the production of neurotransmitters, but may also inactivate catecholamines, precursors of almost all of our good-mood neurotransmitters. The enzyme copper-zinc superoxide dismutase is of enormous importance for the protection of brain cells. This damage-protecting enzyme cannot be synthesized in sufficient amounts when the zinc-to-copper ratio does not favor copper.

Do not worry about copper deficiency. Your daily food contains enough of that trace element. Try zinc tablets for a period of thirty days should you suffer from inexplicable nervousness. They may balance your copper-to-zinc ratio and you may feel better. Also, expose your skin to the bright sun as often as possible to cut down on possible copper overconcentrations.

Secret No. 60

Nervousness is often a matter of zinc deficiency.

Your 30-Day Program for Perfect Nerves and Happy Brain Cells

- *Increase your brain and nerve cell metabolism to 100 percent with the help of your genes.*

- *Be sure to maintain a healthy blood-sugar level—your brain and nerves need glucose.*

- *Take soya-lecithin as a dietary supplement because it contains the precious brain and nerves food, choline.*

- *The amino acid tyrosine is your raw material for more fun and happiness.*

- *Calm your nerves by meditating in nature.*

- *Sleep well with increased melatonin.*

- *Norepinephrine vs. epinephrine—be a winner!*

- *A second reason for more choline is that it is the precursor of concentration and mental alertness.*

- *Take zinc tablets to reduce brain copper; it may also help you relieve your nerve problems.*

MAKE LIFE MORE ATTRACTIVE WITH EXERCISE AND PHYSICAL FITNESS

61 The Fabulous Muscles You Possess

We have about 250 muscles and each of them is a miracle of nature. Managed by neurons, some of our muscles do what we want (like the muscles in our arms or legs). Other muscles do not care what we tell them to do. They are managed and controlled by the vegetative nervous system (like the muscles of our heart or of our digestive system).

Mother Nature differentiates between two types of muscles; Mother Nature would never leave essential muscle movements to our discretion. Involuntary muscle movements include heartbeat and the dilation or constriction of blood vessels or bronchi.

Voluntary muscles, the muscles under our conscious control, allow us limited mobility. In addition, they allow limited physical independence because nature does not want us, for instance, to try to fly—with our extended arms as possible wings. Nature restricts us, as she does with all animals, to our genetic ability. She wants us to remain normal human beings, reproducing, and eating natural foodstuffs. She wants us to stay healthy and happy.

We should not try to pass our genetic limits when it comes to the use of our muscles. Lifting 150-pound weights or tormenting our muscles with all those new and great body-building machines is not what nature originally thought would be our goal. She wants us to stay healthy and vigorous with strong muscles, laugh a lot, and reproduce.

Nature does not expect too much of us. Of course, Mother Nature loves Botticelli paintings, the second set of Mozart's Prague Symphony, and even may admire Stephen King's books. "Look what my human beings can create," she might say. However, physically, she loves to see us with strong muscles.

In addition, nature induces us with a trick to make us love strong muscles. The more powerful our muscles are, the better we feel. We are more dynamic, self-assured, and feel younger.

Isn't that a reason to allow your muscles to use their potential?

Secret No. 61

Powerful muscles increase your zest for life.

62 Tell Me More About My Muscles

Your body weight consists of about 40 percent muscles, assuming that you are in good shape. Your muscle mass consists mainly of proteins, actin, and myosin. They are part of the filaments which make muscle contraction possible. Scientists distinguish between white and red muscles. The white ones contain fewer blood vessels and less of the red muscle myoglobin (that is why they are white). White muscles store less fat or glucose. Sprinters participating in the Olympics 100-meter finals depend on white muscles. These are the sprint muscles, the ones you need when you run to save your child from a dog. Turkeys have white muscles because turkey meat is mostly white. The muscles of a turkey enable powerful and instantaneous flight. This is needed should the turkey be attacked by, let's say, a fox. White muscles are quickly exhausted, but useful for short bursts of energy.

The muscles of a wild duck are dark; they consist mainly of red muscle fibers. The cells of these muscles deposit fat and glucose for energy and also myoglobin which supplies the necessary oxygen for long distance strain. Marathon runners and long-distance swimmers develop up to 80 or even 90 percent red muscles. The way you train your muscles dictates the percentage of red and white muscle. It is not important how you train your muscles, but it is important that you train them. You can make a turkey out of your muscles or a wild duck, but either way would be great.

Muscles need protein to grow. Wouldn't it be great to lose two pounds of fat and gain six pounds in muscle mass?

So, why don't you do it?

It may take you just thirty days, if you take to heart all these brand-new and fascinating discoveries of the genetic researchers or molecular biologists listed in this book.

The dystrophin gene in the chromosomes of our nucleus is the most extended of all of our genes. That is why it takes so long after forty sit-ups to develop new muscle mass. The dystrophin gene is now of immense interest to all athletic coaches, including those of the Santa Monica Track Club. The interest exists because genetic researchers now, in the beginning of the new millennium, lead the way to new training programs—not only for top-performance athletes, but also to us gasping ten-minutes-in-the-evening joggers.

The Dystrophin Gene—Seeing Genetically

❁ *Every one of us has twenty-three pairs of chromosomes in each of his or her roughly seventy trillion cells. Within each pair one chromosome is inherited from Mommy, and the other one from Daddy.*

❁ *A chromosome is an endless long molecule, containing all our genes. This molecule is called deoxyribonucleic acid, abbreviated DNA. All the DNA of a singe cell, nestled together, would be 1.8 meters long. Multiplied with seventy trillion cells, that would mean that you could spool up your DNA strands thousands of times around the sun and earth—an incredible achievement of nature.*

❁ *Visualize these strands as a rope ladder with about three billion rungs. Each rope ladder is then twisted like a spiral staircase and pressed together so that forty-six of them would fit into a microscopically tiny nucleus.*

❁ *About 80,000 active (and about 50,000 inactive) genes extend on this rope ladder, covering or occupying between hundreds, thousands, or hundreds of thousands of rungs. These genes are responsible for the production of happy hormones, of the rhodopsin molecules in our eyes which enable us to see, of synthesizing any one of a thousand different enzymes we need, or of giving rise to the cell division that creates a new offspring.*

❦ *The gene that occupies the most rungs is the dystrophin gene which lets our muscles grow. It extends over three-and-a-half million rungs. When our admired sportsmen or sportswomen have a "bad day," it may because their dystrophin genes were not sufficiently stimulated. Genetic researchers are now becoming the best coaches.*

Secret No. 62

Make a lot out of your dystrophin genes— with just a little bit of physical exercise.

63 More Oxygen Makes You Feel More Adventuresome

Picking up more oxygen by doing exercise in fresh air is the first essential. You should stay outside as often as you can. The best way to invigorate your cells would be to walk through a forest. Trees transform a lot of light energy into chemical energy, releasing oxygen.

No question about it; walking through a forest allows your lungs to breathe in more oxygen than exercising on your ergonomic bike in the basement of your house.

However, inhaling plenty of oxygen does not automatically mean that your muscle cells will be optimally supplied. Every oxygen particle has a rather long way from your lungs into the cells.

Oxygen's Class Excursion

❧ *Your lung alveoli, the pulmonary air cells, have a total surface of about 130 square meters, almost half of what a tennis court has. The inhaled oxygen molecules diffuse through the alveoli right into the red blood cells in extremely-fine capillaries. At the same time, carbon dioxide is moving in the opposite direction.*

❧ *Just a few seconds before, the oxygen particles may still have been within tree leaves. Now they are excitedly rushing into the hemoglobin (the red color pigments) in the red blood cells like a horde of school children on their way to a class excursion. They immediately combine with iron particles. The iron in the hemoglobin is the crucial element for transporting oxygen through the body.*

❧ *The journey begins. Within about eight seconds it leads the oxygen-children through the labyrinth of vessels to all seventy trillion cells. Here they are urgently awaited for energy processes.*

To make a fire or to burn anything, oxygen is needed. In order to burn glucose or fat for energy, our cells need oxygen. The more oxygen that is available, the more cell energy can be produced. That is why a walk in the fresh air, over meadows, or through woods, can be so vitalizing.

Our cells have mitochondria, where fat or glucose is burned for energy. The more oxygen (and other nutrients) that is available, the more mitochondria our cells will create. In addition, it allows more glucose or fat to be transformed into vitalizing body energy. Therefore, the intake of oxygen plays an important role for everyone who wants to be fit and vigorous.

A deficit of oxygen may be the possible cause when someone is chronically fatigued. In addition, a deficit of iron may be the cause because oxygen and iron require each other for energy production.

Secret No. 63

Go out and pick up a load of energy oxygen free of charge— from the trees.

64 Iron Is Crucial for Your Personal Fitness

One of the main purposes of iron is to transport all those oxygen molecules. Iron loves oxygen. The iron atoms hope that there will be sufficient oxygen molecules on their way to the lungs, because just one iron atom can take up one oxygen molecule (which, by the way, consists of two oxygen atoms). Therefore, if there is not enough oxygen coming through the pulmonary alvioli, many of the iron atoms may come away empty-handed. It would be as if it were Christmas and some of the children would get presents and some of them would not. Iron atoms can be very, very disappointed.

On the other hand, the oxygen molecules arrive in the lungs rather concerned; "Will there be enough iron atoms to pick all of us up?" Oxygen and iron love each other so much. Both meet in mitochondrial pathways again, where iron plays an important role for electron transport in aerobic metabolism and where oxygen participates.

Iron may become a problem when you increase your physical activity and fitness program. Athletes, especially runners, often have low iron stores. That may be due to increased blood volume or a decreased intestinal absorption (because digestion may be decreased under stress). Increased iron losses through sweat may be another reason. Excessive exercise may also lead to inner bleeding due to muscle damage and iron loss. Women should keep in mind that they may lose 0.7 milligrams of iron daily through menstrual blood loss.

Many people have an insufficient iron intake due to the lacking of gastric acid. A low pH in the gastric juice is crucial to solubilize and ionize iron. A terrific help is a glass of lemon juice at the beginning of the meal. The vitamin C increases the acidity by stimulating secretion of hydrochloric acid. It promotes iron absorption and it supports iron-dependent metabolism throughout the body.

Iron is not very easily absorbed. Phosphates (in cola, sweet soda, hamburgers, and sausage), phytates (in grain or cereals, spinach, and lentils), and soya products may reduce iron absorption. Tea reduces iron absorption up to 60 percent; coffee up to 40 percent. However, whenever vitamin C-rich food (like fresh fruit) is part of the meal, iron absorption will increase promptly.

Would you like to have enough iron when you start your exercise program? Then eat vitamin C-rich vegetables like cabbage, sauerkraut, tomatoes, potatoes, turnips, cauliflower, broccoli, carrots, pumpkins, Brussels sprouts, or beet roots.

Secret No. 64

Enhance your vitalizing oxygen intake with more iron.

65 Use Your Little Stringent Factors for Better Shape

Not long ago tiny molecules which operate as a kind of warehouse manager were discovered in every cell. They watch and control whatever is coming in the form of nutrients, then they pick up the telephone and inform the managing genes in the nucleus. "We are lacking vitamin B_6," they would announce, or, "There is no more manganese, and threonine (an amino acid) is getting short."

The genes stop the production of proteins the split second not all necessary atoms and molecules are available for synthesis.

This is one of the miracles and mysteries of nature. Nature has never—for billions of years—started the synthesis of a protein or any other substance when not all necessary raw material was readily prepared. This is in much the same manner of a homemaker who tries a recipe out of her new cookbook. She would not start working before all necessary ingredients were laid out on the kitchen table.

It is a miracle because nature has synthesized an almost infinite amount of molecules in billions of years. In addition, not one single second has been wasted in putting together an incomplete substance. It is amazing how these tiny stringent factors cooperate with the genes.

However, what has all that to do with your personal fitness program? It has a lot to do with fitness because when you go out jogging, walking, or swimming, you may reach only 30 percent of the possible success level.

Here is an example: You train for forty minutes with heavy dumbbells in your sports studio. During these forty minutes, your stringent factors tell the muscle-building genes, "Sorry, we do not have any valine or leucine." Both are protein building blocks crucial for the muscles. The genes would stop their transcripts, the pattern matrix, which is necessary for the synthesis of muscle proteins in the muscle cell itself. Messenger ribonucleic acid (mRNA) open new ribosomes, protein factories for more muscle mass. However, if there are no mRNAs, no muscle mass can be produced. You can lift the heaviest dumbbell a thousand times, and it would be useless. Just a few extra muscle fibers would benefit from of all that exertion.

On the other hand, if your cells are well nourished the minute before your training program starts, the genes will send billions of mRNAs into the watery cytosol, the large inner part of your muscle cells. One single muscle cell can now establish up to 200,000 ribosomes for massive protein production and pretty muscle mass. Professional sports people and their coaches will soon use all these new discoveries of scientists. So, why not be ahead of them?

Try it out yourself. Eat a large apple before you go out walking six times around the block or the park. That is what makes your tiny stringent factors happy. In addition, it satisfies the muscle building genes.

Secret No. 65

Don't waste time by doing exercise with badly-nourished muscle cells.

66 How to Build Muscle Mass

Your skeleton muscles consist of muscle tissue, nerves, and tendons. They contain little, if any fat; are mostly pure protein; and besides the connective tissue, are the protein reservoir for our body. That means whenever our metabolism needs amino acids, it takes it out of our connective tissue and our muscles. This is one more reason to cut down on stress (mental stress, for instance) and to get the muscle mass increased.

Warm up before you exercise. It ensures better circulation in muscles and connective tissue so you do not risk getting hurt, which can happen easily, even with negligible exercises. You may incur a ruptured muscle or lumbago with your first sit-up if you do not properly warm up. Avoid overstressing your muscles. Their genes are able to transcript only a certain quantity of the muscle-building mRNAs.

That is, incidentally, the reason why nature created sore muscles. This muscle stiffness originates from tiny muscle fiber ruptures which are caused by lactic acid. Lactic acid builds up when there is too little oxygen available. It may cause pain and tension. You may prevent stiffness by deep breathing during exercise.

You do not need any additional amounts of protein than the ones in your daily food, regardless of the kind of physical training you do. Taking protein supplements from the health store will not help you. Start your exercise program with a limited one-mile walk or jog every day. Very heavy physical exertion in the beginning is more harmful than helpful. There will be stimulation of new muscle mass wherever you put stress on your muscles.

You can double your muscle mass by intensifying your exercise up to endurance training (swimming, biking, or jogging). You will develop better fat utilization, and also store triglycerides (the fat molecules) within your muscles rather than within your belly. Certain genes which manage your fat metabolism, adapt to the new situation when you maintain a regular exercise program. These genes now make fat available in your muscles to avoid the detour from the liver to your adipocytes (the fat cells) and then to your muscles.

When muscles are not trained, they are also insufficiently fed. Untrained muscles develop a poor metabolism, even if your diet contains all the necessary nutrients. In such muscles, the concentrations of water, lipids, and connective tissue are increased in relation to pure muscle mass. Muscles of an untrained person still look stronger than they actually are because they also serve as a glycogen reservoir (the glucose depots). In addition, glycogen has high water-binding properties. That means that the muscle mass of your limbs may even decrease after the first sessions of your exercise program. Do not worry about that. Your muscles will increase their glycogen contents again. In addition, they will develop more muscle mass because of training.

Do not couple an under-caloric diet with muscle exercise. For the building of new muscle mass, protein building blocks (amino acids) are needed. So be sure you need to increase your caloric intake rather than decrease it. Gaining two pounds of new lean muscle mass requires about 6,000 extra calories. Exercise your muscles every day to at least 70 percent of their capacity, even if it is just for a few minutes. In addition, do not start your exercise with abrupt movements. This may increase the risk of injury.

Get yourself a book about less time-consuming exercises such as stretching, aerobics, sit-ups, buttock lifts, leg lifts, knee bends, push-ups, or whatever. Try to find out what your favorite exercise may be. It may be playing tennis, jogging, cycling, swimming, mountaineering, playing volleyball, climbing, or weight lifting.

Secret No. 66

It is fun watching your muscles grow.

67 Water—A Nutrient for Better Fitness

Being vigorous or not is often a matter of how much body fluid you have. Water is the basic element of all that fluid. Dehydration during exercise can cause cramps or weakness. Instead of feeling great, you may suffer from even more fatigue. The vasodilatation of your skin vessels may be responsible. Reacting to exercise-induced heat, they may ooze much blood away in these vessels, resulting in exhaustion or tiredness.

When you lose about 1 percent fluid of what your body weight is, you may be thirsty. Losing more water will bring upon symptoms like mental or physical weakness due to decreased oxygen intake, cardiac output, glucose supply, and other factors. Unfortunately, a progressive water loss is very often not recognized.

Water loss of your body always also means decreased blood volume. Therefore, the blood flow is decreased, and the supply of your cells with necessary nutrients is diminished. Affected is all the electrolyte composition of intracellular and extracellular fluids, which is crucial for vivacity and fitness.

You may ambitiously run five miles, coming home very exhausted. The reason: Heavy sweating has led to excess salt loss. Salt is sodium chloride, and without sodium (and without glucose), water cannot sufficiently enter your cells from the extracellular fluid—which means, your cells are under-supplied and "dry." That is why many athletes take salt tablets in order to maintain healthy body fluid levels during and after practice or competition. An imbalance in your sodium-potassium ratio, due to salt depletion and insufficient fluid supply, may be the cause of muscle cramps.

Water is the best fluid to drink, but you may replace fluid loss with commercial fluid preparations. Your blood volume will increase, and your cells will be better nourished.

Secret No. 67

Try orange juice with a little salt for better success.

68 Learn to Walk Properly

Most of the people in our civilized world do not know how to walk properly. They have lost the ability to move in an optimal way. Natives in the Amazon, the Masai highlands, or the Borneo primeval may not be as skillful as we are in handling a computer-operated washing machine, but they are superior in their way of going or walking.

When we move or carry a load (like shopping bags from the mart across the parking area to our car), we somehow mostly do that wrong. Well, everybody can see that in our streets. We waste too much energy. Members of primitive races develop interplay of muscle power, gravity, and moving force which is more dynamic, effective, and power saving. They also take better care of their tendons, muscles, bones, and joints.

Native people do not often know joint pain, muscle hardening, or stiffening. It is much the same with free-living animals. When we carry two twenty-pound bags from our garage into the kitchen, we do that with significantly increased energy expenditure, wasting a corresponding amount of calories. African or Asian women can carry 25-kilo vegetable baskets or watertanks on their head without frittering away one single extra calorie.

Free-living animals and members of native tribes go in a forward movement, using kinetic energy to push their body forward. The way they move is a steady flexible glide, where movement energy is continuously transmitted into the next step, so it would not get lost.

On the contrary, we walk in an interrupted manner. There is often a short, imperceptible stop when our body reaches its vertical gravity axis, and the kinetic energy is partially lost. We have to push on again and urge our body into the next step. There is an unnecessary energy expenditure, which may lead to earlier exhaustion.

We can learn to walk upright and, therefore, our body gravity rests on the ground. In addition, we need no extra muscle work to prop parts of our body. Practice a type of walking in which you slightly jerk forward, bending the knees. Swimming is an excellent exercise for an upright posture. Another outstanding practice is walking or jogging crossways through a wood because it gets you used to a springy, elastic way of movement, walking over all those roots on the ground. This is also excellent concentration training.

Secret No. 68

Learn to walk like your ancestors.

69) Running Is an Excellent Exercise for all the Muscles in Your Body

Whatever is natural is always the best. So jogging, of course, is a lot more useful for your muscles, tendons, and bones than sports like mountain biking, weight lifting, or tennis. Our body prefers to exercise without the use of sports accessories or athletic implements. Running has been the basic sport for thousands of years.

Jogging not only trains your leg muscles, but every other muscle in your body. In addition, the good thing is that there will be no damage, harm, or injuries to your organism, as there may be with other sports. However, you will have to take a few precautions.

Run on soft and, if possible, warm ground, not on concrete or asphalt. Do warm-ups before you begin to relax tight muscles. First, walk awhile at a brisk pace. Also, do a little stretching after your jogging work-out. You would not believe how many injuries may occur by jogging: ruptures, tearing of ligaments, inflamed joints, and sprained feet. Do not finish your running abruptly but rather end with a short, brisk walk.

Use good running shoes with a well-cushioned sole. Your feet hit the ground often during a three-mile run, so protect them from injury. Also, leave the house for a run when it rains or snows. Cold temperatures increase blood flow and rain may support your cells with more oxygen.

The more you run and the longer distances you run, the more opioid peptides (like beta-endorphin) your metabolism will produce. They are your natural morphine drugs, because they attach to the same cell receptors as cocaine, heroin, or other narcotics. These neuropeptides rise during jogging from a low basal level into blood concentrations where they have an uplifting effect. Many people can't wait to put on their running shoes because jogging is such a wonderful experience.

Secret No. 69

Try running if you are unhappy with your body and mind.

70 Swimming Is the Second Best Exercise

Swimming is the second best exercise possibly because we originally emerged out of the oceans, first in the shape of algae and seaweed, later in the shape of land-crawling animals. However, that was a long time ago. Human beings may have no fins, scales, or gills, but they often feel very comfortable in the water.

That is because water carries us rather effectively. It does not in any way stress our muscles, tendons, ligaments, joints, or bones. Swimming strengthens limp muscles proportionately throughout the entire body. It does not puff the biceps muscles of your upper arm and leave your thighs' muscles piteously meager, as you may experience with one-sided training. Swimming gives you a harmonious body shape. You physically stay the person who you are. This is in contrast to body builders whose body does not conform to their psychological being.

Swimming especially strengthens the muscles of the back and stomach. It gives you a youthful posture. Swimming is the optimal sport for overweight people, because water, particularly salt water, carries well. Overweight people are buoyant because their body fat is lighter than water. Swimming does not place as much stress on the bones of the whole body of an overweight person as other sports do.

Start with short distances to avoid risks. Never swim alone on lakes or rivers, and always keep close to the shore. Also, do not plunge into the water when you are overheated, after a large meal, or after consuming alcohol or drugs.

Secret No. 70

Swimming can be a fascinating new experience for you and your body.

Allow Yourself 30 Days to Change from a Sluggish Weakling to a Vigorous Winner

- *Feed your dystrophin genes. They are the ones which let sportive muscle mass grow.*

- *Supply your organism with more oxygen.*

- *Eat a healthy fruit snack before starting your exercise program.*

- *Iron in your daily meals is crucial for physical fitness.*

- *Do not disappoint the tiny stringent factors in your muscle cells by eating junk food. In that case they would not help you get into better shape.*

- *The build-up of new muscle mass depends on calories, so don't cut down on them with an under-caloric diet or a starvation cure.*

- *Water is an essential nutrient—especially for everyone who does sports and wants to have a powerful body.*

- *Learn to walk properly (which means, above all, upright).*

- *Become enthused about running. It is a physical activity your body will really enjoy.*

- *Go swimming once a week. It will give you a larger lung volume, supplying you with more oxygen when you do other sports—it will also reward you with a youthful body posture.*

THE EXCITING EXPERIENCE OF REGAINING YOUTH: A 30-DAY PROGRAM

71 Becoming Older Has Nothing to Do With Your Wall Calendar

Nature does not comprehend a calendar, your kitchen clock, or the second hand on your wristwatch. Nature has an entirely different understanding of time than we have. For nature, even a trillion years would mean absolutely nothing. In addition, a trillionth of one second, which corresponds to the life span of an oxygen-free radical, does not mean anything to her either.

Time is a creation of human beings. We count sunrises and sunsets, days and nights, and assign numbers. Animals or orchids in a tropical jungle live without the concept of time—free and not under the steady compulsion of a ticking clock and a moving hand. It is fascinating to exist without the regulations of time. Anybody who has been close to nature knows what it is like to be without the sense of time, whether it is on a boat on the ocean or in no man's land, light-years off any road or house.

Living under the pressure of a church tower clock, the car clock, or alarm clock means stress and makes time go faster, accelerating your aging process.

Nature does not care about time. So how does she decide to make a person, a bird, or a plant older? What are nature's criterions to end a lily's life? What about the life span of a zebra or a human being?

The answer is that nature does not know what time is. She does not understand sickness. She also does not know (and does not care) what young or old is; nature strictly distinguishes between healthy and strong cells and worn-out or weak cells. That is because nature "thinks" and acts according to her essentials—very, very simply, as has already been noted in this book. Our cell-life may be extremely complicated, but essential mechanisms (like body weight, aging, and health) are astoundingly simple.

The reason why nature just recognizes healthy or sick cells is that she considers only healthy cells as life worthy. Because, as already pointed out in this book, nature does not want (or actually tolerate) anything weak on her earth. She needed billions of years to develop the earth into a paradise of healthy plants and animals. Nature exclusively, and very urgently, wants healthy plants and creatures to reproduce into new, healthy, and strong generations.

We hold the golden key in our hands—the key to turn back our biological clock.

Secret No. 71

We can become younger and remain young, when we understand how nature expects us to live.

72 Homocysteine Can Make You Older Than You Are

This substance is produced within your body and always tries to make you older. Your cell metabolism fights this substance. Whichever wins will be critical for your aging progress.

Homocysteine is one of nature's two tools to making us older or keeping us younger or of deciding which cells are healthy or not, respectively. The higher your plasma homocysteine levels are, the more you are in risk of mental or physical cell damage. The following chapters will explain how to reduce old-making homocysteine concentrations.

There are twenty different amino acids (protein building blocks) in your daily food. Eight of them are essential, which means that our metabolism is not able to synthesize them from other proteins, so essential amino acids must be in our daily meals. One of them is methionine, which plays a crucial role for your inner biological clock.

Therefore, you had your delicious garlic pasta with shrimp. The "good" methionine will first be metabolized to the "bad" homocysteine. It is very important for your organism to re-synthesize methionine from homocysteine. Because the less methionine is re-synthesized from homocysteine, the more this harmful substance will circulate in your blood.

How Homocysteine May Effect Your Body

- ❃ *Atherosclerosis*
- ❃ *Coronary heart disease*
- ❃ *Systolic hypertension*
- ❃ *Neuropsychiatric abnormalities*
- ❃ *Depression*
- ❃ *Arterial disease, venous thrombosis*
- ❃ *Osteoporosis*
- ❃ *Lack of drive*
- ❃ *Weakness of memory*
- ❃ *Symptoms of old age*

Elevated levels of homocysteine attack practically every single cell. It is nature's tool to test the health of your cells. After that test, nature decides whether to slow or to speed up your aging progress.

Secret No. 72

Homocysteine is the invisible age factor.

73 Why the "Good" Methionine Is of Such Enormous Importance for Your Youthful Complexion

Exciting news now comes from genetic researchers. This is what they explain to us: Between 10,000 and 200,000 protein factories (ribosomes) permanently work in each of our seventy trillion body cells. They produce vital cell proteins. Some of these proteins consist of a mere ten amino acids (the protein building blocks), while others are composed of thousands of amino acids. It takes approximately forty-five seconds to put together such a cell protein. Therefore, using your pocket calculator, you can decide how many proteins are being built in your body within an hour. There are quintillions.

Here is the aging problem: Proteins are like strings of pearls, put together with twenty different amino acids. The first pearl on every such string is a methionine molecule. Genetic researchers call them the initiation codon. On top of each and every quintillion of proteins built within one hour, methionine serves as the locomotive of a long train of amino acids.

This initiation codon will in many cases be cut off from the "amino-acid train" when the protein is completed. The disconnected methionine molecule may then be used again as an initiation codon for another protein. Alternatively, it may be integrated as a regular part of the protein, somewhere in the middle of that "string of pearls." Anyway, proteins can only be built in our cells when there is enough methionine available; that is, methionine re-synthesized from homocysteine.

Cell metabolism will decrease, if there is a lack of methionine in all cells, perhaps dramatically. Ribosomes will close their doors, the cells shrink, and homocysteine concentrations may accumulate in the blood at hazardous levels.

That is the way nature navigates and controls our life, our health, and our youthfulness—with that simple tool of whether or not there will be enough methionine re-synthesized from homocysteine. Sufficient amounts of methionine are equivalent with cell health. Overconcentration of homocysteine means weak cells throughout the body, leading to mental and physical symptoms.

Please read the next secret to learn how to increase your methionine concentrations and to decrease your homocysteine levels.

Secret No. 73

More methionine and less homocysteine are crucial for the quality of your life.

74 How to Crank Up Your Methionine Score

You need three vitamins of the B family to convert more homocysteine into methionine: B_{12}, B_6, and folic acid. People with hyperhomocysteinemia (too much homocysteine in the blood) usually have significantly decreased blood levels of these three vitamins. They are essential for the synthesis of methionine-producing enzymes. Scientists explain us that these enzymes replace a methyl group (chemically: CH_3) into methionine again. Interestingly, they are also the same enzymes which catalyze the ultimate step in biosynthesis of methionine in bacteria. Evolutionarily, bacteria and people from New York, San Diego, Paris, Munich, or London are not so different.

Genetic researchers, molecular biologists, and physicians are now gaining new insights into the progress, diagnosis, and therapy of ailments and diseases. One important result, opening new perspectives into the new millennium, will be the homocysteine-to-methionine-conversion therapy.

You may be ahead of some doctors. Try it out yourself if you suffer from physical or mental ailments. It is so easy, with the help of just three essential vitamins.

– Vitamin B_{12} (cobalamin) is highly concentrated in all kinds of liver (also in liverwurst), cold-water fish, oysters, shrimp, egg yolks, meats, and poultry. Vegetarians may substitute with milk, yogurt, algae, or sauerkraut that will be fermented by B_{12}-producing bacteria in their intestines. The longer someone lives on a strict vegetarian diet, the more perfectly he or she will synthesize their own cobalamin. This, incidentally, explains why people who live traditionally on vegetarian diets (like parts of India or other Asian countries) survive without animal food. However, their grain still contains tiny insects, which deliver enough B_{12}. As a human being, they would not need more than just two, three, or four micrograms of it a day; in their whole life not more than perhaps the size of a lentil. It is a shame, that we kill and destroy all that microbiological life in crop plants with pesticides, so there are no more tiny insects which contributed to the health of people over vast spaces of time during evolution.

– Vitamin B_6 (pyridoxine) is the second crucial vitamin to crank up your methionine levels. It is concentrated in liver, soya or tofu products, nuts, wheat germ, cold-water fish, shrimp, red muscle meats, poultry, bananas (an excellent source), spinach, grains, or avocados. Grain cereals represent a highly recommended breakfast, and are also rich with other precious nutrients. An outstanding nutrition supplement is brewer's yeast or molasses.

– Folic acid is the third of the "Big Three" which may release you from many ailments. It is richly concentrated in liver. Liver is an excellent source of practically all kinds of nutrients, because this organ is the entry and processing workshop of whatever you eat and drink. Dark green salad or vegetables (like broccoli, spinach, Brussels sprouts, cauliflower, chard, and leek) also contain much folic acid. The same is true of lentils, asparagus, soya, grain products, wheat germ, and egg yolks.

In order to substitute corresponding deficiencies, you can take B vitamin-combination drugs, containing all of these crucial nutrients. Do not rely on mono-preparations, like just B_6. Consider all B vitamins as a merry family. They are very sad and listless when separated from one another, and unable to manage anything within our metabolism. This is, incidentally, the reason why nature always puts them together in foodstuffs. Trust them for increasing your possible methionine deficiency.

Secret No. 74

B_{12}, B_6, and folic acid may be the "Big Three" of your new and youthful life.

75 Beware of Free Radicals

Free radicals are, besides homocysteine, the second tool in the hand of Mother Nature. With free radicals, she controls that only healthy creatures and plants forward powerful chromosomes into the next generations. If there were no free radicals, every one of us would live at least 120,000 years. Few people would appreciate living that long.

Nature invented the free radicals at the beginning of evolution, some three or four trillions of years ago. She said to the free radicals, "Listen; all you have to do is just one thing—go out and search for anything that is weak or sick or in any way damaged. Cells, I mean. This will be your one and only job."

"What are we supposed to do when we find a weak or sick cell?" the free radicals asked.

"Try to make it even weaker. Try to destroy it. It is a necessary requirement for the development of a grandiose world that only healthy plants, organisms, and life forms reproduce into in what I call my paradise. You have a responsible task to manage. It is up to you whether my paradise will grow into a great future or not."

Many people think that free radicals are malevolent and naughty, because of what they have either read or were taught on television. In fact, there never has been one single free radical being malicious. Free radicals have an incredibly short life span, some of them surviving no longer than a few trillionths of a second. Within this short period, a newborn free radical glances very ambitiously around, searching for a weak or a sick cell as it was told to do.

In case it would not find one during its short life (perceiving only healthy cells), it would not be annoyed or insulted at all. It would turn off, being bored, at the most. When the free radical finds a weak cell in the neighborhood, it makes a dent into it, but not if it would be caught by an immune substance such as a vitamin E molecule. Even though the radical exists such an unbelievably short time, it still would be recognized by the vitamin E molecule and snatched and neutralized. Yes, these tiny substances show us how to do a job quickly and efficiently.

Free radicals are aggressive substances with an unpaired electron. That is exactly what makes them so dangerous for our cells. Everything on our earth exists of atoms. In addition, pairs of electrons circle atom nuclei. Like couples which love each other and do not want to be separated, electrons do not want to exist alone. Living as a single makes them feel miserable. Therefore, if there was one single electron circling around an atom nucleus, it would jealously watch all the other happy couples of electrons. Finally, it would commit a little offense. It would tear off an electron from the adjacent molecule, now blissfully being part of a couple itself.

However, there is now another single electron, bereaved of its partner. This new single now acts the same; it just steals a single electron from the adjacent molecule. The new single would not wait long to snatch himself another partner—and so it goes on and on, throughout the cell's molecules, at electronic speed. Hit by such a chain reaction, a cell can be destroyed within seconds.

It is crucial for us to protect our cells from free radicals, though they also attack some of our cells' enemies, saving us from diseases. Free radicals develop in our own metabolism, activated, for instance, by junk food or inhaled exhaust fumes. The sun is a potent stimulator of free radicals. Her photons permanently try to invade cells in order to cause damage to them. In addition, the animals and plants must protect their cells from the radicals. In case the plants had no immune protection, it would take the sun's UV beams less than twenty minutes to burn and pulverize all the plants of an entire continent.

Secret No. 75

Free radicals constantly try to make you older than you are.

76 How to Protect Yourself Against Free Radicals

Antioxidants help us protect our cells against these aggressive substances. The better we guard our seventy trillion cells with antioxidants, the longer we will stay young. We can even have our biological clock turn backward again, getting back years the free radicals have robbed from us.

Because every cell is a structure of millions of parts, its metabolism is as busy as the city of Los Angeles. There are different kinds of antioxidants for different purposes in this city life. The four important antioxidants are vitamin A, vitamin C, vitamin E, and selenium.

Vitamin A, in particular, takes care of your mucous membranes by protecting the extremely sensitive mucosa cells from free radicals. Vitamin A keeps off viral, bacterial, and parasitic infections. Vitamin A and its precursors, the carotenes, are considered to have a protective effect against epithelial tumors like bladder or intestine cancer.

The vitamin is a versatile radical scavenger, protecting not only cell proteins and lipids, but also the nucleic acids in the cell nuclei, which are the favorite dish of all free radicals (that way attacking our health from the germ of all cells).

For more vitamin A and carotenoids, eat more green, yellow, orange, and red fruits and vegetables, like apricots, avocado, berries, peaches, melons, pumpkins, broccoli, spinach, tomatoes, carrots, or (one of the best!) all kinds of paprika.

Vitamin C is a powerful antioxidant in all watery cell parts. In addition, because the cytosol, the large inner part of all cells consists mainly of water, you should fill it with vitamin C. This substance is the best companion of vitamin E, by the way. Because whenever a vitamin E molecule is destroyed in the triumphant duel with a free radical, it can be awakened to life again by "Big Brother C," which means by a vitamin C molecule.

For more vitamin C eat fresh fruit (for instance as healthy snacks during the day)—lemons, grapefruit, apples, berries, plums, oranges, cherries, or grapes.

Vitamin E keeps everything lipid healthy. It, in particular, protects the lipid-rich cell membranes and the precious membranes around the cell nucleus, important points of attack for the extremely aggressive oxygen radicals. Endangered by these radicals are unsaturated fatty acids, the ones that are crucial for cell-protecting membranes (especially brain and nerve cell membranes). Plant oils contain much of these sensitive fatty acids. That is why high quality plant oils get very quickly rancid when exposed to light or high temperatures. So dress your salad with a fine olive oil "extra vergine," but never, never (please promise!) fry your French fries with an oil like that.

If you want to build up enviable vitamin E concentrations in your blood and tissue, eat lipid-rich vegetables like avocado, beans, and corn. All kinds of nuts, kernels, and seeds are extremely rich in vitamin E. That is because nature wants to protect these vulnerable "plant babies" from oxygen radicals shot down to earth by the sun.

Selenium is the fourth of the youth-giving antioxidants. Contrary to the other three, this is a trace element. The main purpose of selenium in our body is to be a central part of an enzyme free radicals really do not like at all glutathione peroxidase. This enzyme also neutralizes oxygen radicals, the ones which continually try to get our biological clock hands to move faster. Selenium also builds the most outstanding enzyme in our body, the one that ignites the flame of life within us, thyroxine de-iodinase. The term sounds pretty complicated, however, it is the simplest switch nature has created. It makes tri-iodthyronines out of our thyroid hormone thyroxin (T4)—making seventy trillion cells alive, every day, hour, minute, and second.

Rich in selenium are grain products, natural rice, mushrooms, garlic, asparagus, egg yolk, cheese, fish, shrimp, meats, and liver.

Do you want to stay young? Do you want your cells to be protected from the free radicals? Visit your pharmacy and get yourself a drug with antioxidants. Be sure all four of them are present: vitamin A, vitamin C, vitamin E, and selenium.

Do not give free radicals a chance. Always consider that the cells of an old crocodile look the same as the cells of a young one under the microscope. That is because crocodiles take care of their cells, fighting off free radicals.

So, why not copy them?

Secret No. 76

Stay young (or get even younger) with antioxidants.

77 Nucleotides—The Building Blocks of Youth

Our hereditary disposition is enclosed in nucleic acids. These acids are incorporated into the cell nucleus and are made of nucleotides. They represent the homes of our genes, linking up to form the nucleic acid DNA (deoxyribonucleic acid). As long as our DNA is well guarded, it will manage healthy cell metabolism. When it is damaged and not repaired, it will not properly form our original mental or physical identity. Some examples include our hair gets gray too early, we meet a friend and cannot recall his name, or we develop visual defects.

Scientists explain, that our phenotype has changed by mutations of genes and DNA. Genetic researchers have not noted that such a mutation would have produced a more favorable phenotype—like letting youthful black hair grow again instead of the old gray hair. DNA damage always means bad news.

Our DNA is permanently at risk of becoming damaged by ultraviolet irradiation. DNA is also exposed to the abuse of coffee, cigarettes, alcohol, unhealthful nutrition, drugs, sleep deficiency, lack of physical exercise, and stress. A highly intelligent repair system watches over the health of our genes in every cell in order to keep us young. Special enzymes, called nucleases, recognize the site of damage and cut out the broken part. They then take out their mobile phone and inform special repair enzymes. It takes just a few seconds until the repair enzymes arrive and replace the damaged region.

Our body really makes some efforts to keep us young. Sometimes, however, no repair enzymes appear at the site of damage. "Sorry, we ran out of nucleotides," they would inform the nuclease enzyme through the mobile phone. "Try it again tomorrow."

"Tomorrow it will be too late," the nuclease enzyme would reply. "The damage is in progress. It doesn't look too good."

"I'm really sorry," the answer would be. "You are not the only one calling. We are getting emergency calls from all over the body. All we can hope is that this person will have at least a healthy dinner tonight, with plenty of nucleotides. Lunch was a pizza with coke, two hours later a hot dog with a coke. In addition, some sort of a sweet muffin. Just a miserable few nucleotides came in." The repair enzyme hangs up.

Crucial for staying young or getting younger again is the supply of sufficient nucleotides so your damaged DNA can be immediately repaired and no aging mutations will occur.

Rich in nucleotides are all young foodstuffs like young vegetable and salad leaves—spinach and lamb's lettuce are excellent. Others include beans, peas, lentils, soya, nuts, seeds, kernels, chestnuts, caviar, or eggs.

Secret No. 77

Young food keeps you young.

78 Aging of the Brain

Our brain, even if it is rather small, demands almost 25 percent of all nutrients. That demonstrates that our brain has an enormous capacity and contributes a remarkable portion of the entire cell metabolism.

A baby is born with her or his brain already fairly developed. It rapidly starts to develop dendrites, a rich labyrinth of tender ramifications. Dendrites represent 95 percent of the surface for the contact between neurons. The more dendrite capacity a brain expands, the more receptive power it has.

Within the first hours and days, the reception of a newborn is unbelievable rich. The baby now depends on love, care, and mental activity. Every caress, word, contact, or scent appears to him or her as something amazing. Grabbing at Mommy's cheek is a fascinating experience. A real adventure that is comparable to an adult who for the first time in his life sees Niagara Falls.

That same moment, new dendrites grow and spread out, enriching the brain, making it more intelligent and younger. Therefore, in a way, our brain is the only part of our body, which is able to become younger instead of older. That is why it is so important to keep a baby's brain busy. When a baby is left alone without love, his or her dendrites grow more slowly or temporarily stop spreading out. Mothers in nature never leave their newborns alone. If they are physically alone (when, for instance, the golden eagles parents are miles away, on their way for daily food), they instinctively know that they are not abandoned. "Mom and Dad are still around," the eagle children would happily whisper. They still feel the love and care of the parents.

Dendrites in the child's brain will even die when a baby or a young child receives little or no affection, is treated heartlessly and cold, or undergoes mental and physical punishment. In a case like that, something fascinating occurs: The more parents withdraw love from a child, the more nature jumps in to substitute that love. Nature takes dendrites away from his or her brain or stops the growth of these nervous ramifications. Nature does not want the child to actively seek contact with a hostile world. Nature wants to give the child a chance of existing. Dendrites are another tool for nature to adapt creatures to their environment. A hostile environment decreases intelligence, making the brain "older." A loving environment promotes intelligence, making the brain "younger."

When a baby or a little child is treated cruelly, he or she will often cry. It is a cry for more love. The child instinctively demands for better protection and for extending the brain's capacity. People who have been treated coldly within their early years, need, as an adult, a lot more warmness and caring than people who were raised with love.

Once the brain of an adult is full grown, it has to be kept busy. If it is not it would genetically be adapted to circumstances where less intelligence is needed. Dendrites would die, and the brain's capacity decrease. When dendrites die, their remnants may form amyloids, complexes of dead protein and carbohydrates. Rancid cholesterol and protein garbage will also form lipofuscines. We know those as age spots on our hands. Amyloids and lipofuscines increase the risk of senile dementia (like Alzheimer's disease). That is why it is so important to keep the brain busy, so it would not lose the powerful dendrites. In addition, the good news is that even the brain of an adult can produce new and young dendrites, rejuvenating the brain's capacity.

Train Your Brain

- ❊ *Solve crossword puzzles.*
- ❊ *Play chess or any other game which requires concentration.*
- ❊ *Memorize the multiplication table.*
- ❊ *Learn any text by heart.*
- ❊ *Try to memorize phone numbers rather than writing them down.*
- ❊ *Take soya-lecithin (available in your health store) as a nutrition supplement. It is rich in phosphatidyl-choline, an essential raw material for new brain dendrites.*

Secret No. 78

Your brain dendrites wait for rejuvenating stimuli— take your chance.

79 The Sun Is a Potent Youth Maker

Ultraviolet sunbeams can make your skin old and wrinkled. This constitutes most of the harm the great fireball may do to you.

The sun can make you younger, though. Actually, the sun urgently desires to make you younger. The sun is a friend of nature, though both are close to 100 million miles apart. Three or four trillion years ago, the sun and nature had their first conversation.

"We could establish a paradise on your earth if we stick together. You have the minerals and other stuff. I have the energy," said the sun.

"You couldn't establish a paradise within your fire," nature said.

"And you could not do it with all that dead iron, calcium, copper, aluminum, phosphorus, or sulfur laying uselessly around. Whatever you're so proud of."

So they agreed, and evolution began.

The sunshine-vitamin D acts as a transcription factor in our genes. These factors are crucial for transcript of genes. These transcripts will then be used as patterns for the production of over 50,000 different cell proteins.

There are other transcription factors like vitamin A and the thyroid hormone thyroxine. However, these two factors are dependent on the presence of the major transcription-factor vitamin D.

That was part of the "evolution contract" between nature and the sun. The sun insisted on having lifetime control over nature's paradise. "Because otherwise," the sun argues, "I will help her build up that paradise. In addition, the moment it is completed, I will be off."

Therefore, the photons, the tiny light particles of the sun, control our life from birth to death. The more photons our skin cells receive, the more vitamin D will promote gene transcripts for an increased cell metabolism. That is why vitamin D has an unconditional gate pass through all cell membranes and through the tightly secured inner membrane, which leads to the cell nucleus.

Exposing yourself to light, particularly bright midday light will enhance vital impulses from genes to your entire metabolism. Photons and vitamin D together are great companions as youth-makers.

Secret No. 79

Tap the sun for becoming young.

80 Set Up New Goals

The worst thing which can happen is lacking goals. Genetically, the entire nature's immense combined power is a product of goals—the one achieved, the others not. It does not matter. Goals are great. For a primrose to grow up in spring right into heaven and the sun—what a great goal! For a mole, what a goal—it rhymes! Digging underground tunnels, hundreds and thousands—what a goal! Even for a cloud, traveling to—where?

As our children grow up, they are so enthusiastic about all the possibilities life seems to offer. Never dwell on what already is; life has to keep going on. The moment you insist on what is already established, nature loses its interest in you. On the other hand, the moment you develop new goals (or even just one goal), you are qualified for the ambitious efforts of nature to develop something entirely and excitingly new, whatever it finally may be.

We all know that any good idea can change us. Installing a new kitchen–isn't that a goal? Why not enroll in a yoga class, begin French classes, enroll in that fitness studio, or start with jazz dance? How about playing the violin again or slimming down? Why not plant an herb garden and sell the products? Why not try out for the church choir, move to another state, or perhaps to another country? They want me as an executive manager. Should I accept the job? Are we ready? Should we have another child? Nature kicks in with plenty of energy and euphoria whatever the goal is. It is like a bank which promises to back you with credit money whenever you start a new business.

That is how nature managed it. Nature alone cannot do it. It is a long way to paradise. Nature needs companions who seek the goals—like a dandelion in April which is a thousand times more ambitious than Bill Gates or a squirrel in Vermont which is a thousand times more eager than any politician in Washington.

The moment any plant, creature, or human being sets up a goal, nature would credit that by contributing incredible power. Sure, it is all calculation or computation. However, it is understandable. Whoever lives monotonously satisfied with his or her perfectly mowed lawn, everything under control, would not get that great nature's "goal-and-motivation credit" that can make life so exciting.

Secret No. 80

Goals make you younger.

Nature's 30-Day Program

- *Forget your birth date and your wall calendar. They do not tell you anything about your real age.*

- *Beware of a substance named homocysteine. It attempts to make you old.*

- *Methionine helps you stay young.*

- *Trust in B vitamins: B_{12}, B_6, and folic acid.*

- *Fight off old-making free radicals.*

- *Antioxidants can turn back your biological clock.*

- *Your youthful complexion has its own building blocks—nucleotides.*

- *You may get older, but your brain is getting younger.*

- *Rely on the sunlight. It makes you younger.*

- *Feeling old? What you need is a new goal.*

Your Heart and Your Circulation: Make Them More Powerful

81 What You Should Know About Your Heart

Once upon a time, our ancestors were worms, slithering through the jungle of springtime meadows. They did not need a heart; simple pumping vessels pushed blood through their bodies. When the millenniums went on and on, animals grew bigger and finally human beings walked over the springtime meadows. Our heart now is a powerful four-chamber machine, which operates two circulation systems.

Our heart is the most active muscle in our body. A man's heart weighs about 310 grams; a woman's heart averages 260 grams. The heart beats every minute up to 70 times, forcing about 70 milliliters of blood with every beat into the circulation, about 5 liters of blood a minute. Under stress, it will beat faster (in order to supply our cells with more nutrients through better blood flow). When we go to bed in the evening and turn off the light, our blood pressure will slightly decrease, thus initiating the sleep mechanisms.

The left side of our heart sucks blood out of the lungs, pressing it into the arteries, while the right side forces the blood out of the veins into the lungs, where it will be satiated with oxygen again. Nature has reserved control over our heart. We can influence the heart's work, neither by our will nor by our nervous system, but the heart beats independently, stimulated not by the nervous system but by its own muscle tissue. When an embryo in the womb is growing, its tiny weak heart starts beating though the fetus has not yet developed one single nerve cell. This is something unique, considered one of the most amazing aspects of nature.

Another miracle is that every single heart muscle cell operates its own heartbeat. Certain colonies of such cells are beating imperceptibly faster, giving the beat rhythms, via electrical stimuli, for all other heart muscle cells.

Secret No. 81

Your life-giving heartbreakers are controlled by some miraculous, unknown power.

82 Your Fascinating Circulation

You have about 60,000 miles of blood vessels. Most of them, the capillaries and arterioles, are microscopically thin. The capillaries are nestled among seventy trillion cells. Nutrients such as vitamins, trace elements, and amino acids pass through the vessel walls into the extracellular fluid, from which they are transported into the cells.

The arteries carry the oxygen-rich blood. Connective tissues and muscles strengthen them because the arteries must dilate or contract according to diverse factors. Contraction and dilation are controlled by hormones, or by baro receptors within the vessel walls. These receptors perceive far in advance the slightest changes in the atmospheric pressure. Vessels dilate, and blood pressure slightly decreases when a bad weather front approaches. That can be a calming effect, or may cause one to become even more restless or nervous. Nature slows all her creatures and plants whenever a low-pressure center approaches. This slowing causes dilation of the vessels. Rain falls down and moistens the earth. Plant roots absorb the mineralized water into the widened vessels in order to supply the entire plant. It is the same with the animals or with human beings. Rainy weather is intended for the recovery of the cells.

Our vessels contract when a high-pressure center develops. This slightly increases blood pressure and stimulates us. Stress sets in and muscle tissue around the arteries enable the arteries to adapt to changing circumstances. We should know about this mechanism, because we can manipulate it (as in the case of hypertension). Read about how to do that in the following chapters. Our veins are not strong at all. They are weak and vulnerable with almost no muscle. This is also important, as veins serve as blood depots. This blood reserve is vital should we lose a lot of blood following an injury, or in the case of a woman who is pregnant and needs blood reservoirs for her growing baby. Veins can expand like balloons and hold back more than one liter of blood. This condition does not contribute to proper blood circulation. This happens when veins are undernourished and not well trained (for instance by physical exercise). Read more about varicose veins and other vein problems in the following chapters.

Secret No. 82

Your vessels can be aids in improving physical and mental fitness.

83 Another Miracle: The Blood Flowing Through Your Body

A little more than one half of our blood is watery plasma. This plasma transports the nutrients. The other portion consists of blood cells and platelets which are essential for blood coagulation. The plasma carries about 300 different nutrients or other substances; most of them are amino acids or transport proteins. Our doctor conducts a blood test in order to determine concentrations of hormones, enzymes, white blood cells, vitamins, minerals, fatty acids, and glucose.

There is a large number of cells within our blood. A healthy adult produces approximately 150 billion white blood cells every day—the leucocytes, most of them neutrophils. The bone marrow, a factory creating blood cells, holds fifteen trillion of them in reserve that may be life saving in cases of dangerous virus infections. When viruses invade our tissue en masse, our organism can recruit up to three trillion white blood cells within an hour.

One milliliter blood contains about 4.8 million erythrocytes or red blood cells. Each of them carries up to 250 million of hemoglobin molecules, which gather the life-giving oxygen molecules in the lungs and transport them right into our cells.

Consequently, our blood has a lot of work to do as part of a huge transport system. The blood concentrations of nutrients and other substances change from minute to minute, even from second to second, depending on how much stress we undergo, and the foodstuffs of our last meals. Blood speed is extremely high in the thick aorta—a rate of almost two meters a minute. The smaller the vessels are (within their labyrinthic ramification), the slower the blood flow is. Blood almost comes to a stop when it reaches the very finest capillaries. Here the nutrients are unloaded. After delivering the nutrient load, the blood accelerates again and reaches high speed in thicker vessels. It takes blood substance about eight seconds to be carried throughout the whole body.

There are also enemies in your blood, such as hostile microbes or free radicals. It is crucial to have them controlled by immune substances. Your blood count reflects your general state of health, and as such can be referred to as a calling card of the condition of your health.

Secret No. 83

Better blood count means better health.

84. Something New About Cholesterol

First, there is no "bad" cholesterol. Cholesterol is not only a part of our food, but also produced in our own body as directed by nature. Therefore, it cannot be "bad." Are you trying to cope with cholesterol problems? Then consider this lipid as your friend, not as your enemy. That will make it easier for you to cut down your cholesterol level.

Cholesterol is an essential component of the membranes of all seventy trillion body cells. It also forms hormones, vitamin D, and bile salts. Therefore, it should be obvious that you need cholesterol. Say yes to this lipid. All you have to do is balance your different types of cholesterol—the way you also must balance your calcium-to-phosphorus ratio, your zinc-to-copper ratio, or your sodium-to-potassium ratio. There are always antagonists in our body. Your organism is a composite of substances, which balance each other out. It is the same with the hormones, the enzymes, or between the immune system and hostile particles or microbes.

Within an hour after a meal, cholesterol concentrations in your blood increase. Your cells love that because they need the lipid substance. What is considered "bad" cholesterol molecules, the LDL, travel enthusiastically and ambitiously throughout your vessel system in order to make your cells happy and healthy.

The liver joyfully watches the game. The liver loves making human beings healthy. The liver watches the "bad" LDL entering cells. After a while, it receives a signal that the cells have obtained their sufficient LDL portions. The liver then sends out another substance to bring the excess LDL back to it.

These pick-up transporters are the HDL-cholesterol molecules, often considered as "good," although there is not any "good" or "bad" cholesterol. HDL molecules swarm out into the blood labyrinth, take their brothers and sisters, the LDLs, by the hand and take them back to the liver. There the LDLs are modified to bile substances and secreted into the gallbladder. Everything within our body is arranged in perfect order.

Sorry to say, however, sometimes there are no, or too few, HDL pick-up trucks. That makes the LDL-cholesterol molecules very sad. They consider it as senseless to circulate through the blood-vessel system, for hours, days, weeks, or even longer. All they want is to get home to the liver. It is as if kids were being abandoned. Instead of being picked up by the brother-and-sister HDLs, they must recognize that even more LDLs accumulate.

When fewer HDLs are dispatched from the liver to pick up the LDLs, the more HDL receptors on the liver-cell membranes decrease in number. This makes the situation worse, often even hazardous because the liver cells say, "Why do we need entrance doors for them if there are no HDLs?" That means that LDL cholesterol accumulates while the ability to withdraw them from blood circulation is seriously diminished.

This is the situation of people with cholesterol problems. They should fight their problem from two sides:

1) Cut down on cholesterol-rich food such as all animal fats with their saturated fats, also the hidden ones in hamburgers and hot dogs. The skin of fried chicken is the worst cholesterol bomb. Avoid refined carbohydrates such as pasta, pizza, and white bread. Moreover, leave the sugar where it belongs—on the supermarket shelf. Your metabolism also makes cholesterol out of sweet and refined food. Substitute with whole grain products and vegetable oils and fats which do not contain cholesterol. Avocados are very good as substitutes.

2) Give your liver the chance to build more HDL pick-ups again. Lecithin, particularly soya lecithin with high concentrations of phosphatidyl-choline, is an excellent nutrition supplement. This substance is essential for the coating of many new HDLs. Vitamin C is also very important for a decrease in cholesterol

levels. Make it a habit to eat fresh fruit as a snack against hunger attacks. A fruit breakfast is the best way to start a cholesterol-fighting day. Two hours later you will become hungry (a good sign!), and then you can eat a whole grain slice of bread with a little butter, cheese (cottage cheese is the best), meager meat, smoked salmon, or chicken meat without the skin.

Secret No. 84

Become a friend, not an enemy, of your cholesterol.

85 Hypertension and Atherosclerosis

Take the water hose in your garden and turn on the water. The water will feebly dribble out. Narrow the opening and you will see that the water will shoot out because of the high pressure. Your blood pressure operates in much the same manner. When vessels, particularly the arteries, narrow, the blood pressure increases. Atherosclerosis leads to narrowed vessels—and consequently hypertension. Actually, it is one of the main causes of hypertension.

The endothel, the sensitive inner film of the arteries, can be weakened by a deficiency of important nutrients. In addition, stress requires enormous amounts of protein, minerals, or vitamins. This film now becomes vulnerable. It may easily be damaged by different factors, for instance by homocysteine (a harmful molecule already described in this book). The vessel wall responds with different cellular alterations once there are tiny fissures in the endothelial layer.

Blood coagulates in order to tighten the fissure. Fibrin, a blood clotting factor, accumulates. The metabolism of certain saccharides (sugar substances) falls out of balance. Muscle and connective tissue cells proliferate, producing increased collagen. Blood proteins and oxidized cholesterol stick to that accumulation of substances. Finally, calcium joins the party, building crystals and strengthening the developing vault. The artery narrows and the blood pressure increases. Moreover, bacteria use this necrotic and lipid outgrowth to settle in. This bacterial invasion aggravates the illness.

A common warning sign is heavy pain under the breastbone, sometimes accompanied by pain in the left arm and by profuse perspiration. A heart attack, a cardiac infarction, may occur—a rupture of heart capillaries under the immense pressure of the heart muscle's power. Then parts of the heart tissue will become necrotic in very short time—a hazardous, life-threatening situation. Such ruptures and bleedings can also occur in the brain, leading to a stroke.

It is very important to lower the blood pressure. Above all, substitute salt with spices and herbs. Salt is sodium chloride, the sodium part binding much water. Therefore, the blood volume and the blood pressure will increase after a salt-rich meal. You will also realize that by diminished micturition, or the urge to pass water. Sodium also increases the tension of the vessel walls, contracting the arteries and increasing the blood pressure even more. All kinds of vegetables and legumes are rich in potassium, which is a natural antagonist of sodium, draining water out of the body and dilating vessels.

Moderate endurance sports like bicycling, walking, and swimming help lower the blood pressure. Sports such as weight lifting, climbing, or sprints may, however, be harmful. Try to reduce stress. It stimulates adrenergic receptors on cells, which contribute to a high blood pressure. Lose weight if you weigh more than you should. There is a significant relationship between hypertension and obesity. The heart must work harder to supply the extra body tissue with blood and nutrients. Obesity also favors the development of diabetes, which is an additional risk factor for high blood pressure. Smoking contracts vessels, thereby increasing blood pressure.

Secret No. 85

Vegetables and rest are the best companions on the way to a lower blood pressure.

86 Hypotension: When Blood Pressure Is Too Low

Fatigue, giddiness, lack of drive, nervousness, cold extremities, and vertigo are possible symptoms when the systolic blood pressure sags under the index mark of 110 for men and 100 for women. The larger of the two numbers in your blood pressure test represents the maximal systolic pressure.

Hypotension is not as hazardous as hypertension. However, it also presents risks, such as a tendency towards collapsing or palpitating. Sometimes people with low blood pressure are very unhappy. They have the feeling of lacking something other people have. Sometimes they have the feeling of not being totally involved in life—it is like someone sitting aside, watching other people always having the fun.

Nevertheless, people with low blood pressure may hold an important advantage. Their blood pressure may rise from a low basal level to a somewhat higher index, stimulating the sympathetic nervous system which heightens one's alertness and concentration. This may indicate a predisposition to creativity. It is no wonder that many great artists, show business people, or even sportsmen suffer from a low blood pressure, but during work, performance, or competition their blood pressure rises and stimulates a rich network of hormones and neurotransmitters.

As you can see, there is not much to be concerned about by having low blood pressure. Men and women with low blood pressure often do not have sleeping problems like people with hypertension. In fact, hypotension may easily be controlled or elevated, at least temporarily. Affected people are advised to use more salt in their food. The sodium in salt binds water and increases the blood volume, which leads to a slightly higher blood pressure. Salt also increases the tension of blood vessels, contracting arteries and veins, so that the blood pressure is additionally stimulated. Free-living animals sometimes develop an instinctive urge for salt, when their blood pressure does not match physiological levels. Then animals wander for miles to find salt stones to replenish their salt supply.

People with hypotension should consume more fluid (water, tea, and fruit juice) because drinking raises the blood volume and the blood pressure, particularly that of people with hypotension.

Sometimes, the affected person feels an inexplicable weakness, often before noon or in the afternoon. Respectively water deficiency or blood volume deficiency may trigger this. Eating something salty and drinking a big glass of mineral water may chase off the weakness within five or ten minutes. An excellent drink for people with hypotension is salty vegetable juice.

Also recommended are cold showers or leaving the house lightly dressed, slightly freezing, and walking or jogging vigorously to warm up. Physical exercise and activity can also be very helpful.

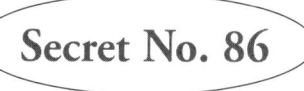

Secret No. 86

Salt and fluid may be beneficial.

87 Why Do So Many People Neglect Their Veins?

Narrowing is the artery's main problem. The vein's main problem is widening. Veins can easily be stretched because they are only slightly reinforced by connective tissue and muscles. Their thin walls become even thinner and more porous. Blood can then penetrate through the pores in the wall. More precisely, weak vein walls may act like a coffee filter through which the liquid components of the blood can penetrate. This is the yellowish-white blood plasma.

Consequences of such extravasations are edemas, particularly above the knuckles, but also in other parts of the body, such as above the wrists or under the eyes. Another symptom may be excessive sweating because the body tries to get rid of water accumulations within the tissue. Excessive water is usually eliminated through the kidneys and the bladder. Weak veins cause some confusion within the body. Affected people suffer from strangury and other micturation problems caused by insufficient urine flow. As further consequences, the bladder and urethra may become infected by bacteria and inflamed. In addition, candida yeast can invade descending urine tracts.

The reason of all that mess is that people do not treat their veins properly. All they have to do is strengthen and tighten the vein walls—and nourish them well. Veins need particularly two substances: vitamin C and rutin, a bioflavonoid. Both are substances which fortify the vessels in plants. We eat these plants and they enter our body in order to tighten the vessels (which, of course, is just one of their many responsibilities). The more inhospitable an environment is for plants, the more rutin they concentrate in their vessel walls. It is therefore not surprising that buckwheat is rich in rutin. Buckwheat is viable under conditions where other plants no longer exist, for instance in the Russian tundra or the Andes highlands.

Rutin and other vein-tightening bioflavonoids are concentrated not only in buckwheat, but also in citrus fruits, fruits, black currants, and other red, blue, or dark berries. Bioflavonoids in the form of combination drugs or rutin as a single drug are available at pharmacies and health stores. Vitamin C is concentrated in all types of fruits and in vegetables.

Walking strengthens the veins, whereas standing damages them. Physical exercise, in combination with vitamin C and bioflavonoid-rich food, is something your veins love.

Secret No. 87

Exercise, rutin, and vitamin C help tighten your veins.

88 No One Must Have Varicose Veins

Varicose veins develop when vein walls are thin and weak and pressure is placed upon them. This occurs when working in an upright position all day or by being overweight (during pregnancy, for instance). Most affected are leg veins, because pressure impairs a sufficient return flow of blood up the legs to the heart. Certain vein walls, which control this backflow, do not close sufficiently, and venous blood is bogged down in little vessel bags and chambers. These vaultings line up and form the ugly, extremely undesirable varicose veins. Little ruptures of thigh or lower leg veins lead to unwelcome bruises.

When veins are plugged, the venous blood searches for detours and bypasses on its way back to the heart, so much of the blood, which would ordinarily flow through skin near the leg veins, now finds its way through inner veins. That means that a lot of venous blood would not participate in circulation anymore, being bogged down in dead veins. This lifeless blood, gathered in sometimes large crevices, can make up to one liter in volume. That deteriorates the capacity of circulation and impairs the nutrient supply of all cells.

Moreover, the alarm bells ring in our organism, because veins are in danger of being ruptured. So plenty of clotting factors will head for the affected vein regions to eventually tighten them. One of them is fibrin, which concentrates in the tissue around the varicose vein. Rancid, oxidized fat and cholesterol substances join it. The fibrinolytic activity of the body is decreased and the risk of a thrombus formation increased, when veins are in danger of becoming completely blocked. The accumulation of fibrin and fat hardens, leading to the unsightly, inflexible yellow leg regions, which are meandered by blue- and red-elevated-vein worms.

Recovery of veins comes out of the intestine with the help of fibrinolytic food. The active agents allium sativum and capsicum in garlic, onions, all kinds of pepper, paprika, chili, and leek activate the blood flow and dissolve fibrin-stimulated blood clotting. Keep in mind, whatever is hot and spicy is good for your veins. This also includes herbs, mustard, ginger, horseradish, radish, or chives.

Try to relieve your legs and elevate them while resting. Exercise helps a lot to get the "dead" blood in your legs flowing and the vein valves functioning again.

Secret No. 88

Veins like it hot.

89 Activate Your Blood Flow

Please read secret No. 88 in the previous chapter to discover what kinds of foodstuffs stimulate your circulation by fibrinolytic activity. Some other foodstuffs contribute by increasing the blood volume and by nourishing all organs and tissue, which participate in the blood's circulation, like the heart or the vessels.

All hot and spicy plants, often containing alkaloids, have been nature's drug hundreds of millions of years before human beings dared to take the first steps into this paradise. Nature made the red pepper spicy in order to protect it against hostile microbes, parasites, and bacteria and against other enemies like birds, snakes, insects, and bugs. A robin or a rose chafer does not like its meals so hotly seasoned.

On the other hand, when free living animals become ill (because they have an infection or because their blood flows too slowly), they instinctively search for the hot stuff that might burn the ailment out of their body. It is no surprise that hot and spicy food has been used for thousands of years as a cure for all types of illnesses.

One of the best drugs out of nature's fantastic pharmacy is vinegar. When an apple or a grape falls to the ground, the sugar within will ferment and be converted to alcohol. After a while, perhaps after some days, vinegar bacteria will convert the alcohol to vinegar. There is a very specific reason: Mother Nature values nothing more than chromosomes and genes, because they carry forth the genus into always new generations. Mother Nature does not care a lot about the fruit pulp, in fact. The fruit pulp just serves for nourishing the seed or kernel, so that another apple tree or vine may grow out of it.

Now comes the reason why nature created vinegar. When an apple or a grape lies on the ground with the pulp decaying, everybody wants to take advantage of it. Birds with their sharp beaks, mice with their sharp teeth, insects, ants, bugs, worms, threadworms, flies—and even the tiniest animals of them all, bacteria, viruses, parasites, fungi, and other hostile microbes—attempt to use the spoiled fruit. Nature makes the vinegar in the pulp more acidic each day in order to frighten off the greedy little animals and in order to save the precious seeds or kernels.

For thousands of years, the acid components of vinegar have been the best household remedies for better circulation. In fact, our grandmothers and grand-grandmothers used to warn, "Vinegar destroys the blood, it makes the blood too watery." It is true, what they said. Unfortunately, those were times when not everybody had a refrigerator. Foodstuffs like vegetables, eggs, mushrooms, or meat were preserved by vinegar in order to feed the family through long winters, for instance. Therefore, people consumed vinegar in quantities which were not healthy.

What we should do, and what is healthy, is to use more vinegar for salad dressing or for spicing. Ketchup, some chutneys, marinades, mayonnaise, and mustards also contain vinegar. Pickled onions, cucumbers, beans, tomatoes, carrots, garlic, shallots, cauliflower, mushrooms, even pumpkin, or plums should be eaten to stimulate blood flow.

Secret No. 89

Vinegar is the best stimulation for your blood flow.

90 Additional Ways to Help Your Circulation

Cold showers are potent stimulators of blood flow. That is because the sudden cold on roughly two-and-a-half square meters of bare skin awakes your circulation. An enormous amount of warm blood flows into the skin cells to beat back the intruding cold. The same holds true for hot/cold showers and with the sauna, which is nothing but an extended hot/cold shower to your body.

Physical exercise also gets your blood flow going and the more you exercise the better. Your cells attain a higher metabolism when you follow a proper exercise regime. Running, bicycling, walking, swimming, and stretching activate the circulation for better nutrient supply. By doing sports, especially the muscles and the heart require increased blood supply to be optimally supplied with oxygen, vitamins, minerals, proteins, and other nutrients.

Substitute saturated animal fats with omega-3-fatty acids in fish or plants (like avocado). These fatty acids are also very effective as fibrinolytic agents, blocking blood platelets from sticking together. It is well documented that people who consume large amounts of fish, like any coast dweller, rarely develop heart attacks or venous thromboses.

Secret No. 90

Rely on cold showers and the omega-power.

A Fabulous Circulation in Just 30 Days

- *Use your blood vessels as tools for mental and physical fitness.*
- *Healthy food will improve your blood count two hours after the meal.*
- *Solve your cholesterol problem with a little bit more understanding.*
- *Vegetables, fruit, sleep, and rest are excellent weapons to fight hypertension.*
- *The best weapons for people with hypotension (the low blood pressure) are salt and fluid.*
- *Tighten weak and porous veins with vitamin C and rutin.*
- *Hot, spicy foods and vinegar get your circulation going. They are great ways to avoid venous disease, varicose veins, and bruises.*
- *Want to do even more for better blood flow? Try omega-3 oils in plants and fish, cold or hot/cold showers, and physical exercise.*

THE WONDERLAND OF OUR ORGANS AND OUR DIGESTION

91 Health and Your Intestines

Our mouth, stomach, and intestines constitute the large entrance hall for all food. Nutrients such as water, vitamins, trace elements, minerals, fatty acids, amino acids (the protein building blocks), and glucose (the building block of carbohydrates) are dispatched by the intestines. These nutrients determine our mental and physical well being. The healthier our food is and the better we break it down, the better nourished our seventy trillion cells will be. In short: your health is directly related to the health of your intestines. It is very easy to establish it, but difficult to regain it.

Our intestines can be compared to the roots of a tree. The only real difference is that it happens that we can walk on two feet. Nevertheless, the food we eat and drink should still be natural, after the model of the tree, which takes natural substances out of the earth. Soft drinks and sodas, hamburgers, microwave food, hot dogs, and candies are not natural foods. It is not the kind of food our intestines expects. Now consider that you have disappointed your intestines year after year, decade after decade—what a shame—how cold and unloving it is!

Not only your intestines, but all of your organs often so desperately try to make you healthy. You would not believe how happy your intestines and your cells are when the remnants of a rich dish of uncooked vegetarian food arrive in your intestines.

Secret No. 91

Our digestive system can be so unbelievably delighted by healthy, natural food.

92 Your Stomach Is a Heavy Worker

The food we eat is not very easy to dissolve. We realize that by cooking. We can boil meat for hours and hours, even the whole day, and the amino acids within it will still be held together. However, it is crucial to breakdown all food into its tiniest building blocks as quickly as possible. That is why the stomach produces gastric acid to disintegrate the food components. Gastric acid is hydrochloric acid. The gastric acid of a healthy man or woman is so acidic that it would burn a hole in your carpet.

So you may consider what kind of acid attacks your stomach wall has to beat back. Actually, healthy mucous membranes of the stomach wall do not get in contact with the gastric acid because the mucous membrane is rather thick and its inner layer is covered with alkaline mucus. In addition, we all know from our chemistry lessons in school that alkaline neutralizes acid. Again it is always astounding, how innovative nature is.

Our stomach has a rather long shape. Its gastric acid concentrations vary considerably. In the upper region, enzymes digest mainly carbohydrates. The farther the food pap descends, the more acidic the gastric juice because in the lower regions, the protein components of food are pre-digested.

There is one other extremely important function of gastric acid—killing all the harmful bacteria, parasites, fungi, viruses, and other hostile microorganisms in food. You cannot imagine how some foodstuffs appear under the microscope, teeming with quadrillions and quadrillions of those microbes. They almost burst with ambition to cross the acid barrier of the stomach, because once they are through, they arrive in the more alkaline milieu of the intestinal digestive juices. Here they would say, "Oh, it's absolutely great here—it is a paradise.

It is warm, moist, and dark in here, so nobody can discover us. And there is a permanent supply of food, out of mysterious reasons."

The bacteria and other microbes will then settle down and develop into mighty colonies, and it may be very difficult to ever get rid of them again. They would not become less ambitious, now trying to invade other parts of the body, through the mucous membrane and via the blood.

The dilemma of many people over 35 years of age is that they produce too little gastric acid with the tendency of producing less the older they get. The best thing to do is to drink a little lemon juice or apple vinegar (dissolved in water) before the main meals. These drinks stimulate cells in the mucous membrane of the stomach to produce large quantities of hydrochloric acid. This is, incidentally, the reason why people in southern countries traditionally squirt a little lemon juice over their fish. They have been doing that for thousands of years. It is not because the fish tastes better, as we might believe, but because they know that the protein in the meal will then be better broken down.

Secret No. 92

Help your digestion with a little lemon juice or apple vinegar.

93 Your Intestine Is a Lush Amazon Jungle

Under a microscope, the mucous membrane of a healthy intestine appears like the Amazon jungle. There are numerous tiny tufts called villi, that are cracks or furrows that allow the intestine to cover a larger surface. If the intestinal wall of a healthy person could be laid out, it would have the surface area of a tennis court.

In case this person would eat a fine blueberry pancake, the mush of it would spread over that immense surface like a wafer-thin film. This enables every nutrition molecule to get in contact with the mucous membrane and slip through it into the bloodstream.

Enzymes of the pancreas, like protease for protein, amylase for carbohydrates, and lipase for fat, do the rest of the digestion work. While carbohydrates are easier digested, proteins must absolutely be degraded to their little building blocks, the amino acids. Predigestion by gastric acid is a first essential for that; now there must also be sufficient quantities of proteases. If someone lacks gastric acid and his pancreas is not working sufficiently, proteins will not be entirely degraded. They will reach lower regions of the intestines and start decaying, with the consequences of indigestion like diarrhea, flatulence, or obstipation.

What is even worse is the amino acid supply of seventy trillion body cells is insufficient. The cell metabolism decreases, and the affected person would feel chronically fatigued, nervous, or even timid. Being undernourished with amino acids, the organism devours them out of the own connective tissue, which may then break down.

The disaster begins. Large, unbroken protein molecules press through the mucous membrane into the blood. They will be considered as intruders by immune substances, which start fighting them—often with allergic reactions. The blood tries to drive out the useless and superfluous proteins through the skin—with the possible effect of acne, eczema, and other skin problems.

Poor Trace Elements

❖ *Vitamins are nature's treasures because they can make dead trace elements or minerals, the moment they connect with these atoms to form co-enzymes. That is why vitamins are quickly transferred out of the food into the blood and to the cells.*

❖ *It is more difficult with the trace elements like selenium, manganese, copper, zinc, iron, vanadium, chromium, iodine, fluorine, silicon, boron, and others. What they urgently need are tiny protein ships or carriers. Trace elements cannot pass the mucous membrane by themselves. They need amino acids to jump into and to be carried through the blood vessel labyrinth to all cells. That is another reason why it is so extremely important to degrade proteins into amino acids.*

❖ *When there are no tiny protein boats, the trace elements are very, very sad and broken hearted. "Why aren't there any ships?" they would ask. "We are waiting here in the upper intestine, but there aren't any ships to carry us to the cells." In addition, they would sadly continue, "It was so wonderful, so marvelous, when we were playing metabolism with our brothers and sisters, the vitamins, just one hour ago, in that spinach leaf. Now all the vitamins are waiting for us in this person's cells, wishing to continue playing with us. But there aren't any small ships to bring us there."*

❖ *Then something disastrous will occur—all the precious trace elements will be excreted with the stool. In addition, the affected person will not only suffer from immense protein deficiency, but from ailments and illnesses caused by a lack of trace elements.*

Secret No. 93

Pamper your intestines with healthy food— and they will coddle you with mental and physical fitness.

94 When Cells Are Hungry

The intestines love vegetables as well as potatoes, grain products, natural rice, salad, legumes, and mushrooms. When it is well fed, its mucous membrane grows exuberantly like the Amazon jungle. When the intestines are badly fed with refined, sweet, or fat junk food, the mucous membrane will rather quickly thin out and lose weight.

The epithelial cells, which form the inner membrane layer, have a short life of only a few days. They are then shed off and replaced by new ones. A healthy intestine may easily shed 200 grams of worn-out epithelial cells daily. This mass will then be digested itself; what ever is a useless remnant will be excreted.

You can ruin the mucous membrane of your intestinal wall within two or three weeks by living on the previously mentioned miserable food, such as drinking too much coffee and alcohol, smoking cigarettes, and taking drugs. On the other side, you can build up your personal Amazon jungle by eating healthy food over the period of a couple of weeks. When a pathologist holds a piece of colon in his hands, it will be heavy when it is healthy, and piteously light when the former owner had been living on junk food. Parts of the epithelial layer may have horns and be dead, increasing the risk of colon cancer and other diseases. Even if a patient with an intestine like that would consequently live on healthy nutrition, the capacity of the mucous membrane would be dramatically diminished, and just a rather small percentage of vitamins, trace elements, and other nutrients would reach the blood.

At nine o'clock in the morning, the body cells have a look at their wristwatches and say, "Let us see what he had for breakfast today." When the blood arrives with fresh nutrients, they would place their order. The blood may reply, "I'm sorry, but we have no manganese today, neither do we carry vitamin B_6, magnesium, or the amino acid methionine at the moment. All I can give you is plenty of sodium and some vitamin A, selenium, calcium, and copper. The poor crumbs of iron I have already promised to the heart cells."

The body cells would respond with untold disappointment. "How can that be? We try so eagerly to keep this man mentally and physically fit. In addition, he feeds us with lousy alms of nutrients, day after day." During the whole day they keep lamenting, "We need nutrients! We need nutrients." And the blood would answer: "I'm sorry, but for lunch he just had a hot dog and a slice of pizza with a Coke again. And in the afternoon one muffin and some ice cream."

The metabolism, manager of all body cells, would shrug his shoulders in resignation. In addition, sometime the cells would also resign, saying, "Forget about it. It is useless with this guy."

That may be the moment when cells die and the biological clock accelerates. The age process progresses as if in a time lapse.

Secret No. 94

Allow your cells proper meals when they need them.

95 Your Liver: The Fabulous Factory Within You

Our liver weighs approximately one-and-a-half kilos, is the body's largest gland and inner organ, and is located in the upper right area of our abdomen. The liver is an incomparable factory; its employees are quadrillions of enzymes which work twenty-four hours a day. In relative comparison to a gigantic company like General Motors, our liver would be a million times more productive. The difference is that our liver does not build cars but essential substances for our organism (like bile, for instance). In addition, it serves as a depot for glucose, protein, vitamins, and many other substances.

That is why there is an enormous blood flow through the liver, about 30 percent of the blood coming from the arteries and the rest from the portal vein which carries noxious substances. The liver works as a detoxifying and cleansing organ. It cleans the blood of the toxic substances, which are produced and absorbed from the intestines.

The hepatocytes, the tiny liver cells, are extremely sensitive. That is why they must be regenerated or replaced because a nonfunctional liver would lead to severe illnesses within a short time. Our liver cells are aware of what is happening in this modern world with unhealthy food and pollution of the environment. They prefer that our daily food may be as healthy as the food our ancestors used to eat. The liver craves clean food, growing out of healthy soil. All drugs, cigarettes, coffee, alcohol, and too much fat are hostile enemies to our liver cells. Hepatocytes are frightened by these substances because they are so vulnerable and defenseless. They are like babies, helplessly yearning for their mother's affection.

Secret No. 95

Consider your liver cells as babies who are yearning for your loving care.

96 Something New About Your Kidneys

Their main job is to filter the blood, to excrete harmful or useless substances, and to give the good ones back to the circulation. Our organism appears to be very complicated, but the important mechanisms function in an astoundingly simple way. Fluid and water enter with the food and are used to wash metabolic garbage out of the body. The moment this body fluid leaves the kidneys heading for the bladder, it becomes urine.

To take care of this important task, our kidneys are provided with two million tiny filters called nephrons. Within each of these filters, there is a control unit, which has a thorough check on all that fluid passing by. "No, we don't need vitamin C at the moment, nor B_2, chromium, phenylalanine, phosphorus, and sodium," someone says. "Give it to the bladder. Retain iron, zinc, vitamin K, magnesium, and potassium. Also the amino acids glycine and leucine." That way the kidney headquarters permanently try to establish physiologically correct blood concentrations.

The kidneys are rather small, weighing no more than about 160 grams. They produce the urine, fixing it up with a certain acidity. This is important for killing all the damaging bacteria, fungi, and other pathogenic microbes, which creep up the urethra (women are, understandably, more endangered than men). The kidneys also regulate the total water volume in the body and they manage the acid-base balance of the blood. The kidneys also produce some hormones, which are needed for calcium metabolism, the synthesis of red blood cells, and other purposes.

Consuming too much protein food can build up toxic concentrations of urea in the blood, because the minute kidney nephrons are not able to get rid of it. Urea easily crystallizes in long prisms; beautiful under the microscope but not so welcomed by joints, wherein this nitrogen-containing substance can cause painful ailments. Gout is a good example of that.

In every hour the kidneys control about eighteen gallons of flowing blood. They need and love a permanent fluid flow, which keeps them functioning, and capable of washing out substances that are not only harmful to the body but also to the kidneys themselves. Because the efficiency of the kidneys decreases during aging, older people should drink more.

Secret No. 96

Help your kidneys: Cut back on meat and drink more water.

97 Your Poor Pancreas

This is the most modest of all organs, never complaining or hurting. Every teacher in the world knows them—those little girls or boys, who are always dutiful and reliable, never obtrusive nor attracting attention. The pancreas is less than 16 to 20 centimeters and weighs around 70 to 80 grams.

The pancreas is not in the service business like the blood, for instance. It is a producing workshop of various products—every day more than a liter of high quality digestive juice with alkaline (non-acid) reaction. Other high-tech products in the pancreas catalog are digesting enzymes like proteases for protein, lipases for fat, amylases for carbohydrates, and nucleases for nucleic acids (the ones needed for formation of genes and chromosomes). What makes the pancreas particularly essential is the synthesis of two hormones which keep (or should keep) your blood sugar concentration on a healthy level, insulin and glucagon.

Your pancreas will secrete insulin into the digestive juice when you eat carbohydrates. This is done to transport the degraded glucose into cells. Your blood sugar rises when you eat a muffin. Insulin transports the blood sugar, the glucose, into the cells and the blood sugar level will fall.

However, our body, especially brain and nerves, are very thankful seeing good concentrations of glucose in the blood. So whenever the blood sugar level falls under a certain line, they will cry out for their energy food.

Like a good mother, the pancreas will immediately produce and send off its other hormone, glucagon. This one will run to the liver and open glucose depots, glycogen the scientists call them, and plenty of glucose will fill the blood again; the level rises.

For many hundreds of million years, the pancreases of animals (there were not any human beings yet) lived a peaceful life. Then came sugar—the one in the sugar bowl, that is. In addition, refined carbohydrates showed up in noodles, sandwiches, pizza, hamburgers, and all kinds of cakes and cookies. That meant a permanent alert for the poor pancreas.

One bagel is consumed, and billions of insulin molecules rush out into the blood. Level rises, falls, alert bells ring again, forcing the poor little gland to synthesize glucagon molecules en masse. Blood sugar goes up, making brain and nerves viable again.

There it goes, the pancreas never getting to rest. However, where other organs complain with pain (for instance), like the heart or the stomach, the pancreas humbly keeps working, never complaining, never hurting. This goes on for years, in fact for decades.

Then, finally, it is too late. There are no harmless pancreas ailments (like heart burn for a stomach ailment or itching for a skin ailment). There are no warning symptoms.

There are people who never complain about being sick.

"Cancer," the doctor may say. Pancreas cancer belongs to the most lethal types of cancer.

Secret No. 97

No more sugar, no more refined carbohydrates—give your poor pancreas a chance.

98 Make a Fortress Out of Your Immune System

It is very true: Nature's conception is incredibly simple wherever essentials are affected. The plainest of them all characterizes the balance between stress and immune system.

Every thought, every minute movement means stress, just as heavy physical activity or a fierce and passionate emotional outburst (either in love or in conflict) means stress. So whatever we do is stressful—driving a car, playing golf, studying the new discount offers of the adjacent supermarket, doing the spring cleaning, falling in love (which is a lot of stress), even falling asleep. Every kind of stress, either negligible or massive, is an attack on our body cells. Stress weakens these cells—as long as they are not protected by a strong immune system.

There is stress everywhere caused by bacteria, virulent substances, and mental or physical pain. Digesting food is stress as well as excreting the remnants. Even being hungry means stress. Enthusiastically planning the next summer vacation is stress as well as lifting Grandma's one ton heavy wardrobe from the basement up to the attic. In every case stress immediately attacks the cells.

Protecting the cells against stress attacks is crucial for the survival not only of us human beings, but also of all major and minor animals and plants. As long as stress cannot be harmful to cells, we will stay young and healthy. That is why we should avoid stress, under any circumstances which is beyond our strength—alternatively, beyond the power of our immune system. In that case, our immune system is not capable anymore of protecting our cells. The immune system will be, as a consequence, vulnerable and defenseless against free radicals, bacteria, viruses, and other harmful substances and influences.

Our immune system is a complex structure, consisting of four important components:

1) The thymus gland is the center of the immune system. It produces a certain type of white blood cells, the lymphocytes or killer cells which are the nightmare of hostile bacteria, fungi, yeast, viruses, parasites, and other microorganisms. The thymus gland has a tendency to shrink when we get older, then it has to be well nourished and protected by vitamin C (in fresh fruit), vitamin E (in plant oils), selenium and zinc (in whole grain), and beta-carotene (in all dark green, yellow, and red fruits and vegetables). Highly recommended for recovery of a weakened thymus gland is an antioxidant preparation, containing the vitamins A, C, and E, plus the trace element selenium.

2) White blood cells are the police officers within the immune system force. They fall into different groups like neutrophils, eosinophils, basophils, monocytes, or lymphocytes, all of them powerful enemies of all hostile intruders as well. Virtually all trace elements, vitamins, and other nutrients are essential for the functioning of the white blood cells. That is why healthy nutrition is so crucial for our mind and our body.

3) The spleen is the superb cleansing system. Weighing between 150 and 200 grams, it destroys and replaces worn-out or damaged blood and immune cells, which engulf and destroy foreign particles and substances. The spleen also produces lymphocytes.

4) The lymph is a bright-yellowish fluid; it is nothing else than the blood plasma, the watery part of our blood. It leaves the minute capillaries and gathers as interstitial fluid or lymph, when it flows through lymphatic vessels. The lymph collects toxic and pathogenic substances and particles and takes them to the lymph nodes, where they are destroyed.

The liver and all mucous membranes in our body also participate in the network of our immune system.

Secret No. 98

Your immune system needs rest, too.

99 Instinct: What We Can Learn from Animals and Plants

Plants, even the unsightly weed by the curb, can be proud of having a hundred times more sensitive hormones than we have. In the late night, when our eyes register nothing than darkness, plants already detect the first photons, sunbeams from the sun. Plants "know" exactly what is going on around them.

They don't have eyes and they don't have ears, but they perceive by instinct what kind of other plants are growing too close to them or what kind of insects are approaching them, so they might secrete some defense poison. Plants are aware of temperature changes by the thousandth part of a degree.

They own sensitiveness which is far ahead of ours.

Free-living animals view their world with incredible alertness. They are always wide awake, steered by an instinct which is, in every second, effected by thousands and thousands of single sensual impressions. When a cat strolls through a harvested cornfield, searching for a mole or at least for a fine vole, it involuntarily perceives hundreds of noises (wind rustling, a bird chipping, an insect buzzing), visual impressions, odors, or scents. The cat lives in a fascinating, exciting, and thrilling world. Never would it like to reverse roles with us.

Our babies and growing kids still live in this adventurous environment. The older we get, the more we are regulated by norms and standards which take care of us, making instinct superfluous, even undesired. That way we voluntarily disclaim a proper portion of living quality. Genetically, we are capable of viewing the world as exciting and breath taking as all the plants and free-living animals do.

What can we do?
- Remember to keep an eye open for the minute, seemingly negligible things, like the fine petal of a daisy, the cute little legs of a ladybug, or the golden-green sparkling of a star.
- Discover the variety of tastes and flavors in vegetables again. You may be held captive by the same tastes, salty-fat or sweet.
- Enjoy the scents of herbs; use them in your kitchen.
- Listen to what nature tells you—the manifold songs of the wind, the murmur of the spring, and the crackle of the ground of the forest.
- Discover the changing light by sunset and the changing forms and colors of trees or bushes when the daylight fades away. Try to describe what you see. Try to experience a walk over a stubbled-field the way a cat might experience it, with all of those hundreds and hundreds of fascinating impressions.
- Develop more curiosity for your environment, and for the people who live around you.

Secret No. 99

Open your genetic floodgates for more emotions and instinct.

The Way to Healthy Organs and Perfect Digestion

- Your digestion system loves natural, unrefined food.

- Try a little lemon juice or apple vinegar right before your main meals. It may do miracles for your mental and physical condition.

- Feed your cells the way you want to be fed yourself— with the best food nature offers.

- Your fantastic liver cells are yearning for a little better understanding and treatment.

- Just half a liter of more fluid a day will keep your kidneys in terrific shape.

- Live without sugar and refined carbohydrates— for the sake of your pancreas.

- Make a fortress out of your immune system.

- Improve life quality with better emotions and finer tuned instincts.

THE GREAT AND NOVEL NUTRITION PLAN FOR THE NEW MILLENIUM

30 DAYS TO HAPPINESS, BEAUTY, AND HEALTH

JOIN THE PROMISING PLUS-30 PROGRAM

It is so easy:
Live strictly on 30 healthy foods
and suspend the 30 "bad" foods.

Hands Off These 30 "Bad Boys"

White bread and bagels
Sugar
Cakes, cookies, sweet pastries, and pies
Sweets and candies
Ice cream and fudge
Puddings and sweet cremes
Pasta and refined grain foods
Refined, polished white rice
French fries
Instant meals and microwave food
Canned foods
Foodstuffs containing too many preservatives
Sausage and hot dogs
Fat bacon or ham
Fat meat
Poultry skin
Liver (more than two servings a week)
Ground beef
Hamburgers or other burgers (except vegetable burgers)
Pizza
Fat mayonnaise, dressings, and dips
Fat, salty sauces
Grilled or barbecued food
Breaded meat
Potato chips and salty fried crisps
Coffee (more than two cups a day)
Liquors
Sweet wine and liqueur
Sweet drinks, soda pops, and cola
Too much salt

Help Yourself With These Good 30

Fruits
Salads
Vegetables
Legumes
Mushrooms
Potatoes
Natural rice
Whole grain products (like noodles)
Eggs
Milk
Cheese and curd
Yogurt
Butter
Plant oils
Nuts, seeds, kernels, and chestnuts
Fish
Shrimps, prawns, and lobster
Meager meat
Poultry (without the skin, sorry)
Wild game and venison
Meager bacon or ham
Tofu products
Seasonings, spices and herbs, and vinegar
Honey
Dried fruits
Whole grain bread, toast or crispbread, and pumpernickel
Cereals
Water and mineral water
Black tea and herbal tea
Fruit and vegetable juices

10 Recommended Breakfasts

1) Whole grain cereal with fruit pieces, nuts, seeds, and cream, sweetened with honey, molasses, or sweet orange juice

2) Pumpernickel with butter, roast beef or cold meat, gherkin, coffee or tea

3) Whole grain bagel with butter, 1 hard-boiled egg, 1 small tomato, 10 olives, goat or sheep cheese, cucumber slices, caraway, coffee or tea

4) One banana mixed into one glass of warm or hot milk, molasses or honey as sweetener, one tablespoon of sunflower seeds

5) Whole grain toast, butter, green cheese or curd, coffee or tea

6) One ripe avocado (Cut it into two halves, take out the pit, splash with a little lemon juice, pepper it, and eat it with a spoon), coffee or tea

7) Whole grain bread, butter, shrimp, one piece of pineapple, mango pieces, coffee or tea

8) Whole grain bread, butter, two scrambled eggs, tomato slices, salt, pepper, and orange juice

9) Fried chicken liver (in butter), salt, whole grain toast, coffee or tea

10) Whole grain bagel, butter, smoked salmon, dill, coffee or tea

Recommended Lunch Ingredients

Main protein dishes
  Cold water fish like mackerel, halibut, salmon, herring, codfish, trout, or any other fish
  Shrimps, prawns, lobster
  Meager meat such as veal, beefsteak, mutton, lamb, liver, kidneys
  Wild game, venison
  Chicken, duck, goose, turkey
  Tofu products

Vitamin and mineral donors
  Spinach, broccoli, beet greens, carrots, black salsify, cabbage, artichokes, asparagus, eggplant, cauliflower, Brussels sprouts, collards, chard, leeks, peas, beans, lentils, kohlrabi, tomatoes, pumpkin, radish, celery, sauerkraut, turnips, kale, onions, garlic, paprika, mushrooms, and all salad greens like endive, lamb's lettuce, chicory, garden and iceberg lettuce

Carbohydrate garnishings
  Potatoes, wild or natural rice, yams, corn, sweet potatoes, polenta, and whole grain pasta

10 Recommended Dinners

1) Uncooked vegetarian food with hard-boiled egg, tuna, and pumpernickel

2) Smoked trout filet with horseradish, whole grain bread, and butter

3) Small veal chop with natural rice, fried tomato, and buttermilk

4) Baked potato with green cheese

5) Fried tofu pieces in spicy cream sauce, whole grain toast, and butter

6) Whole grain bread with butter, tartar seasoned with onion, gherkin, salt, pepper, and paprika

7) Whole grain pies with honey curd

8) Mozzarella with tomatoes (both sliced), basil, vinegar, plant oil, and whole grain bagel

9) Tomato-corn salad with onion and parsley; yogurt sauce with sour cream, lemon juice, salt, and pepper; and whole grain toast with butter

10) Grilled fish with lemon slice, a colorful fresh salad, Italian dressing, and wild rice

The Healthiest Snacks

Nuts, seeds, kernels, and chestnuts

Dry fruits

Banana

Melon slice with meager bacon and crispbread

Tomato filled with green cheese, and whole grain toast

Pumpernickel, one sliced hard-boiled egg, and fat-free mayonnaise

A cup of apple rice, sweetened with honey

Bean salad with small pieces of cold meat, onion, and whole grain toast

Colorful fruit salad with cream

Grated carrots with plant oil, lemon juice, salt, pepper, chopped parsley, whole grain toast, and butter

Curd with grated apple, cinnamon, and honey

Whole grain bread with butter, sliced radish, salt, and chives

INDEX

A
acid-base balance 235
adipocytes 18, 102, 106, 117, 118
adrenal medulla 144
alveolar bone 56, 94, 98
Alzheimer's disease 146, 194
amylase 71, 228
antioxidants 188, 200
apple vinegar 16, 30, 46, 66, 72, 81, 138, 227, 244
arterial disease 179
arteries 179
arthritis 82, 93
ascorbic acid 17
atherosclerosis 179, 211

B
bacteria 32, 39, 49, 95, 97, 99, 182, 211, 215, 219, 226, 235, 239
bacterial plaque 99
biotin 39, 42, 51, 65
bladder 80, 188, 215, 235
blood circulation 45, 205, 208
blood pressure 202, 204, 211, 213
blood sugar 118, 120, 237
blood vessels 13, 32, 82, 94, 99, 104, 108, 152, 204, 214, 222
blood-brain barrier 142
bone loss 90
bones 13, 61, 78, 80, 87, 92, 168, 172
brain 14, 114, 126, 128, 130, 133, 140, 142, 146, 184, 191, 212, 237
bruises 217, 222

C
candida yeast 215
capillaries 99, 157, 204, 211, 240
carbohydrates 61, 97, 102, 130, 209, 226, 238, 244
cardiac infarction 211
cardiac output 166
carotenes 24, 188
cartilage 92
catecholamines 148
cavities 95, 98
cell metabolism 10, 13, 42, 45, 84, 113, 150, 178, 191, 197, 228
cellulite 12, 18
cholesterol 41, 84, 87, 110, 134, 194, 208, 211, 222
choline 134, 138, 146, 195, 209
chromium 229, 235
chromosomes 9, 41, 56, 58, 155, 185, 219, 237
circulation 26, 45, 140, 144, 163, 202, 209, 217, 221, 235
cobalamin 182
collagen 13, 15, 22, 24, 26, 115, 211
colon 231
copper 61, 66, 148, 150, 196, 208, 229, 233
coronary heart disease 179
carbohydrates 61, 71, 97, 102, 104, 130, 194, 209, 224, 228, 238, 244
crow's feet 12

D
dandruff 67
dentine 94
depression 179
diabetics 130
diarrhea 16, 228
digestion 72, 99, 138, 140, 226, 228, 244
dopamine 66, 136, 138

E

elastin fibers 12, 14
enamel 94, 97
endorphins 137
enzymes 10, 41, 43, 49, 65, 106, 139, 148, 155, 182, 191, 226, 223, 233
epidermis 12, 28, 32, 35, 37, 40, 71
epinephrine 62, 144, 150
epithelial cells 231
erythrocytes 69, 206
estrogen 86

F

fat 18, 32, 46, 71, 84, 102, 108, 116, 118, 154, 163, 217, 231, 233, 237, 243
fatty acids 26, 61, 71, 134, 189, 206, 221, 224
fibrin 211, 217
filaments 154
flatulence 16, 228
fluorides 98
folic acid 65, 148, 182, 200
follicle glands 32
free radicals 24, 37, 63, 75, 92, 99, 113, 185, 188, 200, 207, 239
fungi 33, 48, 95, 220, 226, 235, 240

G

gastric acid 16, 65, 71, 82, 111, 138
genes 9, 13, 41, 56, 58, 69, 113, 126, 133, 150, 161, 163, 174, 191, 196, 219, 237
gingivitis 99
glucagon 62, 237
glucose 26, 39, 61, 71, 96, 112, 118, 130, 142, 150, 158, 164, 206, 233, 237
glycogen 114, 130, 164, 237
growth hormone 108, 110, 124
gums 22, 99

H

heart 14, 56, 120, 139, 150, 154, 195, 202, 211, 217, 221, 232, 238
heart attack 211
homocysteine 178, 180, 182, 185, 200, 211
hormones 45, 62, 81, 93, 108, 110, 112, 126, 134, 144, 155, 208, 213, 235, 237, 242
hypertension 179, 204, 211, 213
hypoglycemia 130
hypotension 213, 222
hypothalamus 112

I

immune system 20, 26, 47, 208, 239, 240, 242
inflammations 35, 92
insulin 118, 124, 130, 237
insulin receptors 118
intestine 71, 80, 82, 84, 105, 106, 111, 116, 130, 182, 188, 218, 224, 226, 228, 231
iodine 112, 122, 229
iron 61, 69, 73, 81, 82, 114, 157, 159, 172, 196, 229, 235

J

joints 82, 92, 100, 168, 170, 236

K

keratin 36, 54, 61
kidneys 14, 80, 82, 84, 115, 215, 235, 244

L

leucocytes 206
libido 140
linoleic acid 61
lipase 71, 106, 228

253

lipofuscines 194
lipogenesis 102
lipolysis 102
liver 14, 25, 39, 61, 66, 104, 106, 114, 116, 146, 164, 182, 208, 233, 237
lymph 32, 240
lymphocytes 35, 240

M

magnesium 80, 82, 231, 235
manganese 161, 229, 231
mediators 47, 92
melanin 43
melanocytes 43, 56, 59
melatonin 142, 150
menopause 86, 98
menstruation 86
metabolism 10, 13, 16, 27, 35, 42, 45, 47, 71, 82, 90, 114, 116, 121, 142, 159, 163, 170, 178, 180, 183, 193, 228, 229, 235
microbes 33, 35, 95, 99, 208, 219, 226, 235
mucous membrane 226, 228, 229, 231
muscles 35, 88, 90, 114, 130, 152, 154, 161, 163, 168, 170, 172
myelin sheath 133

N

nerve cells 39, 126, 128, 130, 133, 136, 145
neurons 136, 138, 144, 146, 152, 193
neurotransmitters 45, 134, 136, 137, 148, 213
nicotine 20
nucleases 191, 237
nucleic acids 26, 188, 191, 237

O

obesity 212
obstipation 228
omega-fatty acids 48
oral cavity 95, 97, 100
osteoporosis 86, 90, 179

P

pancreas 65, 71, 118, 131, 228, 237, 244
parasites 33, 95, 219, 226, 240
parasympathetic nervous system 140
periodontal disease 99
phenotype 88, 191
phosphates 134, 160
phosphatidyl-choline 195, 209
phosphorus 78, 80, 82, 84, 94, 98, 196, 208, 235
phytates 160
pigment cells 32
pineal gland 142
pituitary gland 43, 108, 111, 112
platelets 206, 221
polysaccharide 96, 97
potassium 61, 148, 166, 208, 212, 235
protease 71, 228
proteins 16, 45, 54, 94, 98, 109, 112, 118, 128, 134, 154, 161, 178, 180, 188, 196, 206, 211, 221, 228
psoriasis 47, 48, 51
psyche 125
pyrogens 92

R

rhodopsin 155
ribosomes 59, 120, 162, 180
rutin 215, 222

S

saccharides 211
saliva 94, 97, 106
seborrhoa 67
selenium 24, 63, 188, 229, 232, 240
serotonin 142
silicon 229
skin 12, 18, 22, 29, 32, 33, 37, 39, 41, 43, 45, 47, 49, 51, 56, 82, 84, 86, 98, 110, 126, 131, 148, 166, 228
skin inflammation 40
smoking 20, 30, 63, 212, 231
sodium 148, 166, 208, 213, 235
spleen 240
stomach acid 16
sucrose 96, 97
sunburn 43
sweat glands 32
sympathicus 140
symptoms of old age 146, 179

T

tar 20
taurine 37
teeth 9, 56, 80, 84, 94, 98, 99, 100, 219
tendons 163, 168, 170, 172
threonine 161
thymus gland 240
thyroid gland 41, 112
thyroid hormones 112
tissues 12, 13, 16, 20, 22, 24, 29, 78, 84, 84, 94, 98, 110, 114, 204
tooth decay 95, 97
triglycerides 102, 104, 108, 114, 118, 163
tryptophan 142
tyrosine 66, 112, 136, 138, 150

U

urethra 215, 235
UV beams 37, 43, 186

V

vagus nerve 138
valine 161
vanadium 229
varicose vein 205, 217, 221
vegetative nervous system 140, 152
veins 22, 202, 204, 214, 215, 217, 222
viruses 33, 95, 206, 220, 226, 239
vitamin A 24, 41, 61, 63, 73, 188, 196, 232
vitamin B_6 161, 183, 231
vitamin B_{12} 82, 182
vitamin C 17, 20, 22, 30, 61, 63, 88, 99, 110, 138, 159, 188, 210, 215, 222, 235
vitamin D 41, 47, 83, 84, 86, 100, 196, 208
vitamin E 25, 63, 185, 188, 240
vitamin K 83, 235

W

white blood cells 78, 92, 206, 215, 240
wrinkles 12, 20, 82

Y

yeast 35, 183, 215, 240

Z

zinc 17, 22, 30, 61, 66, 73, 148, 206, 229, 235, 240
zinc deficiency 62, 73, 148